THE USE OF DRUGS

THE USE OF DRUGS

Principles of Pharmacology and Therapeutics for Nurses

By
WALTER MODELL, M. D., F.A.C.P.
Associate Professor, Clinical Pharmacology, Cornell University Medical College, and Cornell University New York Hospital School of Nursing

and **DORIS J. PLACE, R. N.,**
Professor of Medical and Surgical Nursing, University of Arkansas, School of Nursing

THIRD EDITION

Springer Science+Business Media, LLC

1 9 5 7

First Edition
First Printing, June 1953
Second Printing, January 1954
Second Edition
First Printing, February 1955
Second Printing (With 1956 Materia Medica), February 1956
Third Edition, June 1957

ISBN 978-3-662-37428-3   ISBN 978-3-662-38180-9 (eBook)
DOI 10.1007/978-3-662-38180-9

Copyright, 1957 Springer Science+Business Media New York
Originally published by Springer Publishing Company Inc. New York 1957
Softcover reprint of the hardcover 3rd edition 1957

Library of Congress Catalog Card Number: 57-10139

PREFACE

We take the gratifying acceptance of two editions of THE USE OF DRUGS to indicate a considerable agreement with its way of introducing students of nursing to pharmacology. Our original contention was that the subject is being taught at many schools in much the same manner in which this textbook presents it and that the book would therefore well fit into such teaching programs; further that its emphasis on principles would be particularly helpful in class room teaching and that its arrangement would also prove useful in continued learning about drugs and in actual nursing.

The character of the book remains unchanged in the present new edition. We have considered seriously and gratefully the suggestions for improvement sent to us by readers. These suggestions and our own second thoughts are now part of the book.

The new Third Edition contains Parts I and II, "Principles," and Part III "The Medicine." "Materia Medica," which formerly was Part IV of the text book, is now available as a separate book only, with the title DRUGS IN CURRENT USE 1957; to remain "current" the small book is being revised and newly dated every year. We believe that the physical separation of materia medica from principles will be helpful for study and in practice.

Since principles are not susceptible to constant change, and new principles are rarely introduced, this book in its present form should not require frequent revision. A chapter on the use of tranquilizers has been added in this Third Edition.

WALTER MODELL, M.D.
DORIS J. PLACE, R.N.

New York, N. Y.
and Little Rock, Arkansas
May, 1957

PREFACE TO THE FIRST EDITION

This book was written for student nurses and nurses as a fresh approach to pharmacology and therapeutics. In presentation and selection of material it emphasizes what the nurse needs to know about drugs and their use. The authors have aimed at making the information easy to understand and easy to find.

Some may take the view that when a nurse measures a drug accurately, presents it to the patient and sees to it that he gets all of it in the manner prescribed, her job of drug administration has been completed. The authors feel strongly that adequate drug administration also implies an understanding of drug actions. The physician shapes the orders but he is present only a small part of the time. The nurse is there all the time and, serving as the doctor's eyes and ears, she should observe the patient and the effects of the drugs she has given him. This is the function which distinguishes the expert nurse. To perform it well she must know what to look for.

All effective drugs are double-edged swords, with a potential for harm as well as a capacity for good. The nurse must be sensitive to both possibilities at all times. If she understands what the doctor hopes to accomplish by his medication and is equally aware of the dangers, she is in the best position to decide, not only when the beneficial effects of the drug are developing but also when something is going wrong; when the earliest signs of drug intoxication appear, when altered circumstances make a useful drug a dangerous one, when a patient is developing resistance, tolerance, addiction or hypersensitivity and when to bring these matters to the attention of the doctor. Her observations, her suspicions and her decisions on the effects of a drug may make the difference between cure and disaster. This kind of information, which is nothing more nor less than the substance of pharmacology and therapeutics, must be a part of a nurse's equipment if she is to give her patient all the benefits which are inherent in good nursing.

The nurse who is well grounded in pharmacology will be better able to adapt herself to the wide differences in the practices of physicians which she may encounter. If she understands the actions of drugs she will also understand why there may be more than one way to treat a disease: she will not be upset when she discovers that two physicians treat the same disease differently and it will not shake her confidence in one therapeutic plan if she recalls a case in which the same illness was treated most successfully in another way.

The picture of drug therapy changes all the time and progress has been swift and revolutionary in recent years. New drugs are being constantly introduced with claims of superiority over drugs already established or with claims for new and novel therapeutic actions. In some cases such new drugs have provided an entirely new approach to treatment or help for an incurable disease. But against a few such miraculous drugs there are many which have not lived up to their promise and are now forgotten.

The physician and the nurse both are likely to be confounded by the large groups of drugs with almost identical actions. In many cases these drugs represent minute variations on the theme of one basic drug, each differing only slightly from the parent drug in actions but differing markedly in the claims made for it by the manufacturer. There are, for example, perhaps 200 derivatives of barbital or veronal. At the head of this long list of barbiturates are drugs officially called phenobarbital, pentobarbital, amobarbital and secobarbital. These are much better known under other and un-official names, luminal, nembutal, amytal and seconal. Each is the favorite of different physicians. Yet the real pharmacologic differences between them are unimportant and each may be used for the same therapeutic purpose with much the same result.

A situation such as this requires stocking medicine shelves with many more drugs than are good for the very best therapy; it com-plicates matters for all concerned, adds to the cost of medication and greatly increases the possibility of error in drug identification. It is a distinct liability and a medical headache.

It is the authors' hope that by giving the nurse a point of view, this book can provide a solution to both the problem of the rapidly changing therapeutic scene and the large number of drugs used. Nothing could be more valuable to the nurse than an approach to drugs in general, as well as an approach to drugs which she has not used before; a way of thinking about drugs, their uses and their dangers.

Although no bibliography is given in this book, the works of others have been consulted freely. Chief among the sources used were the *United States Pharmacopeia* (Mack Publishing Company), *National Formulary* (American Pharmaceutical Association), *Useful Drugs* (Lippincott), *New and Nonofficial Remedies* (Lippincott), Sollmann's *Manual of Pharmacology* (Saunders), Goodman and Gillman's *Pharmacological Basis of Therapeutics* (Macmillan), Howard's *Modern Drug Encyclopedia* (Drug Publications), Douglas' *Formulary and Therapeutic Guide of the New York Hospital* (Appleton-Century-Crofts).

CONTENTS

Part III: The Medicine

Addendum

Materia Medica, which in earlier editions was Part IV of this book, is now
published as a separate book only, with the title DRUGS IN CURRENT USE.

PART I

PRINCIPLES OF
PHARMACOLOGY

1

PURPOSE OF DRUGS

Pharmacology is the basic science of drugs; therapeutics is the practical science of how these drugs are used in the treatment of disease. These are fundamental subjects in the art of healing. Many students approach them with fear and trepidation, thinking them exceedingly difficult to understand. While these subjects can be made to appear complex and bewildering, these are also practical subjects, which for our purposes need not be made more strange or difficult than many everyday matters.

It may be helpful to note that the body handles drugs in much the same way as it handles food. Problems of administration, digestion, absorption, utilization and elimination apply equally and in the same way to both drugs and food. Variations in reactions exist in both cases: some people cannot tolerate certain foods; some people cannot tolerate certain drugs. Similarly, there are problems of overdosage in both: the person who overdoses himself with food gets fat; the one who overdoses himself with drugs gets poisoned.

Every one of you has probably had personal experiences with drugs (aspirin, cathartics and the like) and already made certain observations on their action. Pharmacology is not really an entirely new subject for you. In thinking of how drugs act it is often useful to compare the action of some new drug you give a patient with what you may have seen as the result of drinking liquor, which really contains a drug, alcohol. The effects of alcohol taken for any reason whatsoever are pharmacologic effects just like those of any other drug. The time it takes a drink to produce its effects indicates the rate of absorption of the alcohol from the gastrointestinal tract; the extent of the intoxication indicates how much or how often the dose of alcohol is taken, the length of time the effect lasts is an indication of the rate of elimination of the alcohol;

2

and if the drinker falls all over himself, this is an indication of intoxication by the drug. In this way we observe the effects of drugs on man; later we utilize this knowledge in the treatment of human disease.

Definition

Drugs have been described as all agents capable of affecting living protoplasm. Pharmacology, the science of drugs, is mainly concerned with therapeutic drugs useful in the treatment of disease, and not so much with toxic drugs which are principally harmful or poisonous. Study of the latter constitutes the science of toxicology.

Pharmacology deals with every aspect of drugs: (1) their source, (2) their identification, (3) their physical and chemical properties, (4) their taste, (5) how they may be prepared and stored for use, (6) how they exert their effects on the body, (7) which organ or system of organs in the body they affect, (8) how their effects differ in health and disease, (9) which effects are useful in the treatment of disease, (10) which effects are dangerous or toxic, (11) how the earliest signs of toxicity may be detected, (12) how the drugs may be administered, (13) how the drugs enter the body after administration, (14) the duration of the effects, (15) how the drug is destroyed or eliminated from the body, (16) the safe and effective doses and dosage schedules of the drug, (17) the effect of other drugs on the drug in question, (18) the tendency of the human to develop tolerance, (19) addiction, (20) intolerance or allergies to the drug, (21) how to treat poisoning by the drug.

Purpose

Drugs are used to relieve symptoms, to support and correct disturbed physiologic function and to cure disease. In addition, they are often used to produce an effect on the patient or to produce an effect on a parasite which is causing disease in the patient. In producing an effect on a patient, drugs are used to alter some physiologic function, to depress or to stimulate the activity of some organ or system of organs (the respiratory or cardiovascular system, for instance), or to supply a missing or deficient material such as a vitamin or a hormone. When drugs are used against parasites they may destroy a virus, a bacterium, a spirochete, a mold, an insect or a worm which infests a patient.

In a case of an injury due to an automobile accident the patient may be treated in many ways. If he is in great pain he is given an injection of morphine. This is done solely to produce an effect on the patient, namely to depress his ability to appreciate pain, and thereby to relieve it, but in no way to exert a direct curative action. If the patient is in a state of shock due to trauma and loss of blood he will be given an infusion of plasma. This is supportive treatment; it supplies missing fluid and raises the blood pressure, and in that way supports the failing circulation until the body recovers its ability to do so. Finally, the patient may be given an injection of penicillin. This is given to destroy bacteria which may have contaminated his wounds. If the drug kills these bacteria, it is, in effect, curing the patient of an infection. In this example three approaches to therapy were applied, two of them to produce an effect on the patient and the third to produce an effect on bacteria.

Drugs which cure disease are by far the most dramatic. There were only a few such remedies until twenty years ago, when the sulfonamides and antibiotics (like penicillin) altered the picture and became the drugs of first importance. They have ushered in an era of therapeutic miracles and hopefulness: diseases which used to be fatal are cured, diseases which were marked by frequent and serious complications have been simplified.

Unfortunately, this does not apply to all disease for we have a large number still incurable. Even in those diseases for which we have the miraculous new specifics there still are symptoms to be relieved. Patients must still be treated and cared for. This applies to all patients, especially those for whom there is no medical cure, and since no one is immortal this eventually applies to everyone. The relief of symptoms may be all that medicine and nursing can provide for many who are bound to die. It forms a substantial therapeutic problem as well as a serious burden in nursing care.

The symptom-relieving actions of drugs are, therefore, of vital importance in all patients regardless of the availability of curative drugs or surgery. The restless patient may be rested, the sleepless patient may be given sleep, the uncomfortable patient may be eased, the patient in pain may be relieved of his pain, a sluggish function may be stimulated, an overactive organ may be quieted, a failing function may be supported. Such expectant and supportive treatment not only makes the patient happier—which is still an outstanding part of patient care—but it also enables the body to do a better job of helping itself, and increases the patient's ultimate chances for recovery. The role of relief, rest and comfort in the cure of disease can be ignored no more today than it was in the earliest days of the art of healing when there were no specifics, when all that medicine could offer was symptomatic and supportive treatment.

It must be mentioned here, although it will be repeated later, that every medication given to a conscious patient has yet another therapeutic effect. It provides the patient with reassurance that something is being done for him. This applies to the drugs which cure as well as to those which provide only symptomatic relief and, for that matter, even to those which are without any useful pharmacologic action. Every treatment given to a patient is a symbol which strongly suggests to him that help is being provided. Today more than ever, we recognize the important role of the mind on the body, of psyche on disease and symptoms; when drugs are given, the confidence of the patient that he is being helped also plays a role in events which follow. This important inherent property of all medicaments must always be borne in mind by the nurse. It is a valuable asset of all drugs. Sometimes, unfortunately, it is the only effective modality we can use. It should never be discouraged by the nurse, for she would then be depriving a medication of one of its inherent and traditional properties; it should never be discouraged by an implication of doubt over the effectiveness of the treatment the nurse is administering. On the other hand, such considerations should not lead one to omit more effective drugs.

Study Questions

1. What is the difference between pharmacology and therapeutics?
2. Why are drugs used?

NATURE OF DRUG ACTION

Pharmacologic Action

By definition there is no such thing as drug action without life or without an effect on a living cell; fundamental life processes are involved in all aspects of drug action. The basis of drug action is the effect it has (1) directly on a living cell, (2) on the cell's life activities or (3) on the products of cellular activity. (By cell and cellular activities we generally mean groups of cells, usually large enough to comprise organs, rather than a single cell.) In the first instance a drug may inhibit the essential life processes of the cells of the kidneys and as a result damage or destroy the kidney. In the second instance the drug may act on the cells of the kidney to increase (or decrease) the rate with which it forms urine. In the third case a drug which is excreted unchanged by the kidney into the urine, neutralizes the acid produced by the kidney and changes the reaction of the urine from acid to alkaline.

How drugs enter or affect the individual cells to alter their function is a highly theoretic problem which will not be considered here, but the fact is that some drugs are highly specific in their action and exert profound effects on specific groups of cells without appreciable effects on other cells or organs. Other drugs are far less selective and, if given in effective doses, will have far more diffuse effects on several systems of cells, or organs, of the body.

Sometimes drug action is achieved by direct application of the drug at the site where the effect is desired. For example, a soothing ointment is rubbed directly into an itching area of the skin to provide relief. This is known as a *local* action. In other cases such a direct approach cannot be used, either because the organ cannot be reached by direct application or because the drug must work through some intermediary mechanism. In such a case the drug must be introduced, by one means or another, into the circulation through which it reaches the site of its action. This is known as a *systemic* action. For example, when digitalis is used to produce an effect on the heart, it is taken internally either by mouth or by injection because it cannot be applied directly. In either case the digitalis is absorbed into the bloodstream and finally reaches the heart where it exerts its effects.

Psychologic Action

The above examples of drug action are generally considered to be pharmacologic effects. It has already been pointed out that there is also a psychologic action inherent in all drugs. This cannot be ignored, and because of its importance, will be mentioned repeatedly. Many patients feel better when they get medicine, regardless of its action. For example, a patient may be relieved of her pain by an injection of sterile water. This effect is psychologic, and neither the result of a direct action nor the result of a systemic reaction to the pharmacologically inert water that was injected.

Many patients demand medicine for all their ailments and complaints. Drugs that are given merely to satisfy this desire are called *placebos* ("I please" in Latin). This pleasing action of medicine attaches to all of them, good, bad and indifferent. On the other hand, there are patients, who for equally obscure reasons, are badly affected, psychologically, by all medication. It is not uncommon for such patients to complain that the medications have made them worse in a particular way which clearly could never have resulted from the drug given. Patients resistive to medication in this way must be carefully evaluated; they may increasingly complain although their essential illness is getting better. Both kinds of psychologic effects, the positive and the negative, are so commonly attached to medication that they tend to confuse the evaluation of results. They must always be considered when trying to estimate the true effects of a drug.

Therapeutic and Toxic Effects

A distinction has already been drawn between therapeutic and toxic effects of drugs. Therapeutic effects, in one way or another, are useful in the treatment of disease; toxic effects are harmful. While there are many poisonous drugs which have no therapeutic actions, the reverse does not hold true in the case of therapeutic drugs, for within certain dose ranges, all of them have toxic effects. For this reason it is necessary to be careful in the administration of all effective drugs, for a drug which may save a life in a therapeutic dose, may kill the patient if it is too large. On the other hand, if the dose is too small it may be entirely useless. For a drug to be useful at all, the therapeutic dose must be smaller than the toxic dose.

Therapeutic Range

In some drugs the spread between therapeutic and toxic dose *(therapeutic range)* is relatively narrow; these drugs are difficult to use and require constant vigilance if serious toxic effects are to be avoided. In most of the useful and commonly used drugs, however, the therapeutic range is wide and they may be used with relative safety. Constant observation of the patient is, nonetheless, necessary because individual variations and hypersensitivities may be so great as to overcome the safety factor which the therapeutic range provides for most cases.

Physiologic Basis of Drug Action

When drugs act directly on cells or organs, they either *stimulate* (increase the rate of cellular activity) or *depress* (decrease the rate of cellular activity). With some drugs, there may first be stimulation which is later followed by depression. The ability of a drug to stimulate or to depress a cell or organ depends on (1) the normal function of the organ, (2) the state of health or disease of the organ, (3) the state of activity of the organ. In order to anticipate the effect of a particular drug in a disease these three factors must be considered. Therefore, in all reasonable discussions of drug action and therapeutics the physiology of the several organ systems involved becomes extremely important.

Toxic Symptoms

Therapeutic effects are useful only when they can be obtained with safe and nontoxic doses. Toxic effects are usually distinguished as *minor* or not dangerous, and *major* or dangerous. The former are usually produced by smaller doses and precede the appearance of the latter which are produced by relatively larger doses. In some instances there may be little difference between the doses which produce both minor and major toxic symptoms. Usually, however, the minor toxic symptoms appear some time before the major symptoms and serve as a warning that further use of the drug may have serious effects. For this reason it is just as important for the nurse to know and look for minor toxic symptoms as for the more dramatic major symptoms which are signs of serious damage.

The variety of toxic effects exempts no organ. They may affect the same organ as that on which the therapeutic action is exerted, or they may affect other and unrelated organs. The therapeutic actions of digitalis, for example, are mainly on the heart, but minor toxic symptoms may appear in the gastro-intestinal tract through vomiting. The major toxic effects of digitalis, on the other hand, are manifested in the heart through severe disturbances in cardiac rhythm. In many instances the toxic effect takes the form of serious irritant and destructive actions. For example, chloroform may induce a serious inflammatory reaction in the liver and mercury may induce serious degenerative changes in the kidney. Each of these effects may be fatal.

Study Questions

1. How are therapeutic and toxic effects of drugs related?
2. What factors influence the ability of a drug to stimulate or depress the activity of cells or organs?
3. How are these factors related to the therapeutic use of drugs?

FACTORS MODIFYING DRUG ACTION

The specific effect which drugs exert on certain organs may be altered in both intensity and rate of appearance and disappearance. This variance of drug action may be due to a number of factors not inherent in the drug itself. This chapter, therefore, deals with the following factors which modify drug action: (1) route of administration, (2) rate and degree of absorption, (3) rate of elimination, (4) effect of other drugs, (5) tolerance, (6) idiosyncrasy and allergy, (7) disease.

Route of Administration

The routes of administration are the means by which drugs are applied in order to obtain effects. In order that a drug produce an effect, it must somehow reach the site of its action, the cells on which it acts.

Direct Administration

In some cases it is possible to apply the drug *directly* on some tissue in order to obtain *local* action. The skin, the mucous membranes of the mouth, eyes, nose, pharynx, rectum, vagina, urinary bladder are available for direct application. The *aerosol* spray is a new and novel method of direct application; a fine cloud or *nebula* of solution containing the drug is forced, under moderate pressure, down the respiratory tract, and in that way the drug acts directly on small bronchi.

Oral Administration

In most cases, however, the drug must first get into the bloodstream before it can reach the organ on which it acts. There are a variety of modes of administration which make the drug available for action in or on the body. But the most common and by far the most convenient is the *oral* route. It is also usually the least costly because special preparations are not required. The drug is given by mouth to be absorbed somewhere in the gastro-intestinal tract. When a drug is given in this way, it is subjected to the action of the digestive juices, which may in turn destroy the drug. It is sometimes possible to avoid these effects, however, by coating tablets with a material resistant to gastric acidity (enteric-coating) which does not liberate the drug until the tablet reaches the small intestine.

Other disadvantages of oral administration are found when the drug irritates the stomach or intestine giving rise to nausea, vomiting, loss of appetite or diarrhea. Such reactions may make oral administration impractical. If this is not so, and the drug is absorbed, it will enter the bloodstream from the gastro-intestinal tract in much the same manner as food.

In some instances the drug is completely absorbed and the dose given is totally effective. But absorption is not always complete and in some cases perhaps an insignificant proportion of the amount given will be absorbed into the bloodstream. As a matter of fact, so little may be absorbed as to make oral administration ineffectual. In still other cases absorption may be irregular, sometimes rapid, sometimes slow, sometimes complete, sometimes incomplete. In such cases it is exceedingly difficult to determine the proper dose and another mode of administration may be preferable. Most drugs which are presently used orally, however, are absorbed sufficiently to produce an effect, and enough can be given to compensate for losses due to incomplete absorption. Most of these orally administered drugs are absorbed from the stomach or small intestine, much more rarely from the colon and rectum. In the latter cases they may be given rectally.

Special Routes of Administration

Other surfaces of the body will absorb particular drugs. For example, some drugs like of Oil of Wintergreen (methyl salicylate) are absorbed from the surface of the skin and may be applied that way *(percutaneous)* to produce systemic effects. Some drugs such as nitroglycerin may be absorbed from the cheeks *(buccal)* and under the tongue *(sublingual)*. A few drugs such as the estrogenic hormones are absorbed from the vaginal mucosa *(intravaginal)*. Pituitary extract is effective systemically when applied to the nasal mucosa *(intranasal)*, while the general anesthetics are applied by *inhalation*. There are a limited number of instances in which these special routes of administration for absorption may be used effectively.

Parenteral Administration

The *parenteral* routes avoid the gastro-intestinal tract and provide administration by injection directly into the body. There are many methods of parenteral administration and not all will serve for any one drug. The most direct means of parenteral injection for systemic effects is the *intravenous* injection. Effects come on most rapidly because the drug is injected directly into the bloodstream and there is no problem of absorption. No drug is lost, there is no delay due to absorption and in most cases the effects develop almost instantaneously. On the other hand, it is by far the most dangerous way to administer drugs and serious reactions occur more frequently by this route than by any other. Intravenous injections should always be made very slowly to avoid reactions.

Other methods of parenteral injection for systemic effects require absorption before the drug reaches the bloodstream; that is to say, the injection is made into some tissue and must be absorbed from that site. *Hypodermic* or *subcutaneous* injections are made *under* the skin, *intradermal* injections are made *into* the skin. *Intramuscular* injections are made into the muscle. Effects from these injections develop more slowly than after the intravenous injection, the delay being due to the process of absorption. On the other hand, these modes of administration are safer than the intravenous because the drug does not enter the bloodstream with such rapidity. In some instances the drugs are too irritant to be injected into tissue; severe reactions at the site of injection may result if this is done. In such cases the intravenous route is the only one which may be used for parenteral administration, if indeed, even that route is permissible. Strangely enough, the vein is often able to tolerate far more irritating drugs than the skin or muscle. This may be so because the blood in the vein quickly dilutes the drug and so prevents local reaction.

In cases in which large amounts of fluid must be administered subcutaneously, their absorption may be facilitated by the simultaneous administration of hyaluronidase, an enzymatic material which aids absorption from the subcutaneous tissues by spreading the fluid over a large area.

In infants and small children parenteral administration must sometimes, because of the smallness of the veins, be made into bone marrow *(intramedullary)* or into the peritoneal cavity *(intraperitoneal)*.

Direct applications of drugs may sometimes be made by the parenteral route. Thus in a case of meningitis, antibiotics may be injected directly into the spinal canal *(intrathecal)*. In the same way injections may be made directly into a joint cavity *(intra-articular)* or into the eyeball *(intraorbital)*.

A method of introducing drugs into superficial tissues through the skin by electrical current is *iontophoresis*. The uses of this route of administration are exceedingly limited.

Deciding on the Route of Administration

For systemic action the oral route is always the route of first choice because it is both convenient and safe. Parenteral administration, after due consideration, is the second choice. It is justified in cases in which (1) the drug is not absorbed from the gastrointestinal tract, (2) the drug is destroyed in the stomach or small intestine, (3) the drug is too irritant to the gastro-intestinal tract, (4) the patient is vomiting and cannot retain the drug, (5) effects come on too slowly by the gastro-intestinal route for the particular condition, (6) the patient is noncooperative or unconscious. Thus the state of the patient and his disease as well as the nature of the drug all enter into the decision of how to administer a drug.

Rectal administration may overcome some of the objections to oral administration but, in general, few drugs are well absorbed from the rectum and colon; effects develop very slowly and rectal irritation which is produced by some drugs may be exceedingly disagreeable.

Absorption

Absorption is the process by which the drug is removed from the site of application and enters the bloodstream. The process varies in degree, speed and regularity, each of which has an important bearing on the effect of a dose of a particular drug.

Rate of Absorption

Rapid and almost instantaneous effects are generally produced by drugs given intravenously. Drugs which are absorbed by inhalation may also induce virtually instantaneous effects. Other routes of administration produce effects more slowly. Drugs given by mouth are the slowest to enter the bloodstream and produce effects. This, however, varies greatly with each drug. Some drugs produce effects within as short a period of time as 15 minutes after oral administration; others, such as digitalis, may take 5 or 6 hours to produce appreciable effects. But most drugs lie in an intermediate position. The presence of food in the stomach tends to delay absorption considerably over that on an empty stomach.

Degree of Absorption

Some drugs are completely absorbed from the gastro-intestinal tract so that the dose taken by mouth is equivalent to the amount of drug that enters the bloodstream. Other drugs may not be completely absorbed; in some only as little as 20 per cent of the dose taken by mouth actually gets into the bloodstream. In other cases virtually none is absorbed. Most confusing are those drugs which are irregularly absorbed, in some instances being well absorbed, in others being so poorly absorbed that it is difficult to predict what the effects of a particular dose will be.

Food and Water

Food of all kinds, even milk, tends to delay the absorption of drugs from the stomach and intestine. If rapid action is required it is best to administer oral medication a sufficient period of time before meals so that this interference will not take place. Water, unless very cold, usually has little influence on the rate of absorption and it may be given freely. Very cold water may delay absorption for as long a period of time as it takes the water to warm up in the stomach and intestine.

On the other hand, food sometimes prevents irritation of the gastric and intestinal mucosa by drugs and in some cases symptoms such as nausea, vomiting and loss of appetite may be prevented by giving the drug immediately after meals. In most instances this procedure merely delays but does not prevent the absorption of drugs.

Prolonging Drug Action

There are devices to reduce the frequency of dosage necessary to maintain drug action. They are especially useful and make for grateful patients in the case of parenteral injection. The devices for delaying drug action are of two types: (1) those which slow up elimination and (2) those which delay absorption. In the former, a drug which prevents renal excretion is given together with the drug from which a therapeutic action is sought. This delays excretion and prolongs action. Caronamide may be given together with penicillin to delay with its excretion by the kidneys. Although it was a useful device when introduced, it, and others like it, have been largely given up because of their unphysiologic nature and have been replaced by the devices of the second type, the depot forms. The so-called depot form of medication is an arrangement in which absorption is delayed. A relatively large dose is given and this, together with prolonged slow absorption, produces a persistent drug effect. Well known examples are procaine penicillin and protamine zinc insulin. In the former, the procaine combination slows the absorption of penicillin to such an extent that a single injection may produce therapeutic levels of penicillin in the blood for two or even three days. Doses are, of course, proportionately larger than with the injections of the rapidly absorbed forms of penicillin.

Absorption is an important property of drugs because it relates to the certainty, intensity and rapidity of effects after a dose of a drug. Thus it is important to know about the characteristics of absorption in the case of all drugs one uses.

Development of Action

When a drug is injected intravenously so that problems of absorption are not encountered, the effects usually develop rapidly. In many cases effects may be fully developed in a matter of a minute or even less, as in the case of an injection of epinephrine (adrenalin). This is an example of immediate development of action. In

other cases even though the drug is quickly introduced into the
bloodstream and it reaches the site of its action in an instant, it may
take hours for the full effects to come on. Just what processes are
involved in cases of such delayed action is not clear, but there are
important drugs, like digitoxin, which even after intravenous injection take 5 or 6 hours for full development of effects.

Problems of absorption also delay development of action. Thus
the nature of the development of the action of drugs is a complex
picture depending on variations in absorption as well as in the
development of the drug effect on the cell after it reaches it through
the bloodstream. It is the characteristics of the picture of the development of action of a drug which will determine the situations in
which a particular drug will be used.

Elimination

Once a drug develops its full effect it begins to wane. This
tapering off is due to the elimination of the drug, for if it were not
eliminated from the body its effects would be permanent. Drugs are
eliminated by many different physiologic processes: (1) by the
kidneys into the urine, (2) by the intestine into the feces, (3) by
the liver into the bile, thence into the intestine, (4) by the lungs
into the expired air, (5) by destruction or chemical change *(detoxi-
fication)* in the liver or other organs. Some drugs are eliminated by
one of these processes exclusively, some by more than one. It is of
great importance to understand how drugs are eliminated for one
would hesitate, for example, to give a drug which is eliminated by
the kidneys to a patient with extensive disease of the kidneys.

Rate of Elimination

Drugs vary greatly in the rate at which they are eliminated; some
are rapidly eliminated, as in the case of intravenous epinephrine
which leaves the body in as little as 5 minutes. Other drugs, such as
digitalis, are more slowly eliminated, taking as long as 2 weeks
before total elimination. In some cases blood tests may be used as
an index of the presence of the drug in the body but, in many instances, the drug attaches tenaciously to the cells or organs on which
it acts, and even though little or none may be found in the bloodstream, potent drug actions are still in evidence

The amount of a drug eliminated is usually not a fixed amount in each 24 hours, but rather a per cent of the amount of the drug (varying with each drug) present in the body. Thus when there is very little drug in the body only a small amount is eliminated and when a large amount of the drug is in the body the amount excreted is correspondingly larger.

Knowledge of the rate of elimination is a matter of great practical importance in determining the schedule for prescribing drugs; it is the basis for the decision of how often to repeat a dose in order to maintain effects without causing intoxication.

Cumulation

One of the bugaboos of therapeutics is the concept of cumulation. Both doctors and nurses fear it, yet this fear comes only from a lack of understanding. Most people take cumulation to imply the accumulation, or piling up, of a drug in the body when it is given repeatedly, so that toxic effects are inevitably produced. Drugs are described as being cumulative or noncumulative, implying that the one is far more dangerous than the other. This is not a true picture of the phenomenon for cumulation is more often useful than it is harmful, and it is a source of danger only when approached with ignorance. Cumulation develops when a drug is not completely eliminated before another dose is given. If, in such a case, many doses are repeatedly given the level of drug action in the body tends to rise. What finally happens depends on many factors. In all cases, however, the level of the drug action in the body will eventually stop rising. This will happen when the amount of drug eliminated daily equals the amount of drug which is taken each day. Since, as already mentioned, the amount of drug eliminated daily is not fixed, but a percentage of the amount present in the body, the amount eliminated daily increases as the drug accumulates in the body. Eventually elimination and daily dosage must equate.

The intensity of effects which is finally achieved with the drug depends on the level at which accumulation ceases; that is, when the daily dose taken equals the proportion of drug in the body daily eliminated.

If this is reached below a therapeutic level, even though a process of cumulation has taken place there is not sufficient cumulation to produce therapeutic effects. If the cumulation ceases at a therapeutic level, then therapeutic effects will be maintained by continuation of the same daily dose. If the drug in the body reaches toxic levels, toxicity follows and will intensify until the level is reached. Cumulation will always take place when the daily dose exceeds the amount eliminated daily regardless of the drug used. Where this process ends depends on the level it reaches before the two, intake and output, equal each other. Whether cumulation turns out to be useless, useful or harmful, depends on these factors.

There are many examples of cumulation being used in this way to maintain therapeutic effects after repeated doses. In the case of digitalis, for example, a single daily dose will produce progressively more intense effects until, in the course of about two weeks, full therapeutic effects appear. Thereafter, the same dose continued for years may not alter the intensity of the effects. In the case just cited the digitalis cumulated for two weeks, at which time a therapeutic level was reached. Since the dose was properly adjusted, intake then equalled output and no further cumulation took place even though the same dose was continued long thereafter. A smaller dose of digitalis in this instance would never have cumulated sufficiently to produce therapeutic effects no matter how long continued, while a larger dose would undoubtedly have produced toxic effects in less than two weeks.

Drug Interaction

When a dose of a drug is given before complete elimination of the previous one there is simple *addition* of effects. Addition may also take place in the case of two different drugs with closely similar actions. Thus a dose of digitalis and a dose of ouabain will produce effects which total the separate effects of each. This is so because their effects on the heart are identical. There are instances when the effects of two drugs is greater than the sum of the effect of each. This is known as *synergism*. In this case the action of one drug is to enhance the action of the other. Thus cocaine enhances the effect of epinephrine on the blood pressure. The opposite effect, that of *antagonism*, is much more common than synergism. In this case the action of one drug is to nullify the affects of the other. Thus the action of histamine is eliminated by its antagonist, the antihistaminic drug, pyribenzamine.

Toxicity

Toxic effects create serious limitations to the effective doses of drugs which may be used. Some drugs produce deleterious effects on the bone marrow, some on the kidneys, others on the heart, the brain, etc. The degree to which these organs are endangered, as well as the degree to which they are already diseased, limits the use to which many drugs may be put.

In some cases the dose of the drug which produces the desired therapeutic effects is so close to the toxic dose that there is always serious danger of producing damage to some organ. In other cases the therapeutic dose and the toxic dose are so widely separated that there is relatively little danger of toxic effects from therapeutic doses, and the drug may be considered to be a safe one. In the former example, the drug is often said to have a low *therapeutic index*, which has much the same meaning as a narrow *therapeutic range*, while the latter, and safer, drug is said to have a high therapeutic index or a broad range.

Tolerance

After a drug has been in continuous use the patient may develop a tolerance to it. This implies that a specific dose of the drug produces less effect on the patient than the same dose originally did. Tolerance may develop to any drug, but it develops more quickly and to a far greater extent with some than with others. The mechanisms in the development of tolerance are not clear in most cases, but they can be compared with the increasing ability of some people to drink alcoholic liquors without perceptible effects. When a patient develops tolerance to a drug, progressively large doses must be used in order to produce effects. Since the development of tolerance may not apply to the same extent to the toxic dose, this increase in dosage may bring the therapeutic dose very close to the toxic dose. In addition, the development of tolerance is sometimes closely allied with the development of addiction, and this should be considered in a case of apparent tolerance to addicting drugs.

Addiction

Addiction is a state in which a patient develops a need for the continuation of the drug to such an extent that need for the drug has the same urgency as the need for food or other fundamental drives. This need is usually both physical and psychologic. With addiction the body acquires a physiologic or functional need (as well as a craving) for the drug and serious and disagreeable symptoms may follow the withdrawal of the drug. The best example of this is seen in the morphinist who is suddenly deprived of morphine and suffers severe distress as a consequence. The psychologic addiction usually develops because of the capacity of the drug to produce pleasant effects, dreams or a sense of well being. The craving for this artificially pleasant atmosphere may become exceedingly strong; so strong in many addicts that it becomes the outstanding drive in their lives. Addiction is, of course, much more likely to develop in the case of a drug which produces pleasant effects than in any other type of drug, although exceptions are seen.

Habituation and Dependence

Habituation and dependence are less precise terms than addiction; they are usually applied to a need for the drug which is not so great that social problems arise. Also, withdrawal symptoms are not likely to follow in these cases. The nurse is usually in the best position to detect the beginning of either addiction, habituation or tolerance to drugs. She should bring her suspicions to the attention of the doctor at once.

Idiosyncrasy or Allergy

Idiosyncrasy or allergy represent an extraordinarily high degree of sensitivity to a drug. There is what may be considered a normal range of variation in drug sensitivity, much as one sees in different people's reactions to alcohol; some can take considerably more than others. So it is with drugs that within a broad range some patients require more of a drug than others to produce the therapeutic effect, and conversely, some patients get an effect from far less than others. When this degree of sensitivity is so great that minute amounts produce an intense reaction, a state of hypersensitivity is said to exist. In the case of an allergy this hypersensitivity involves a particular mechanism which is discussed in another section (page 130). In any event, regardless of how the intolerance is designated, when a patient states that he knows that he cannot tolerate ordinary doses of a particular drug, or that he has had an unhappy experience with a drug, this statement should be respected until the physician decides how to handle it. Allergic reactions may be extremely serious and develop with such rapidity as to make it an exceedingly harrowing experience for the nurse.

Effect of Disease

Disease may alter the response to a drug and make one patient react differently from another. Not to belabor this point, it may be pointed out that if a drug is eliminated by the kidneys or destroyed by the liver, and it is given to a patient with liver disease or diseased kidneys, he is apt to handle the drug in a manner quite different from the patient who has normal kidneys to excrete the drug and a normal liver to destroy it. Some diseases alter the nature of drug reaction. Thus a patient with an attack of angina pectoris feels better after a dose of nitroglycerin, while a normal person usually feels very faint and dizzy after a similar dose. In some cases drugs will precipitate disease attacks; for example an attack of asthma may be set off in a patient with asthma by an injection of methacholine (mecholyl) given for some other condition.

Related Drugs

Finally, there are chemical variations in drugs which may alter drug action or modify it to some extent. Modern synthetic chemistry has complicated matters considerably. Whenever a new and useful drug is discovered, chemists immediately get to work and proceed to synthesize a host of closely allied drugs with similar actions. Thus we now have hundreds of barbiturate, sulfa and antihistaminic drugs. These large numbers of allied drugs confuse matters for all concerned, physician, nurse and pharmacist. A nurse may have an experience with one member of a group and not know precisely what to expect when another doctor gives a similar, but not precisely the same, drug to another patient with the same condition.

In general, and there are many exceptions, drugs in the same pharmacologic group tend to have closely similar actions, and to differ quantitatively rather than qualitatively. Thus in the case of two barbiturate drugs used to induce sleep, thiopental and amobarbital, both make the patient sleep in the same way, but thiopental does it far more rapidly; another difference between the two barbiturates is that the patient awakens much sooner after thiopental. More often than not, claims made by the manufacturer for superiority of his product, usually reduced toxicity, are not justified and should be carefully examined before acceptance. The true advantages which related drugs usually have over one another must be determined by the physician; the nurse never is justified in substituting one for the other.

Study Questions

1. What factors may influence the effects and actions of drugs besides their specific actions?

2. Why is it important that the nurse know the means by which drugs are eliminated from the body?

3. What are the hazards and values of cumulation?

4.

DOSAGE

The dose of a drug is the amount which produces a therapeutic effect in the patient without producing dangerous or undesirable side effects. This is a variable amount depending on the potency and pharmacologic properties of the drug, the mode of administration, the patient, his disease, the kind of effect desired, whether treatment is to be long continued and whether the drug is a particularly dangerous one. Unless all of these are considered, the dose chosen for a particular case may have no meaning, may be ineffective or may be dangerously large.

Potency of Drugs

Molecule for molecule, some drugs are far more potent than others. The effective dose of nitroglycerin, for example, is usually about 0.5 milligram, while the effective dose of urea may be as large as 15 grams, 30,000 times as large.

In each range of potency, however, the drug has a toxic as well as a therapeutic dose. Thus when the average dose of a particular drug is a fraction of a milligram, the toxic dose usually is in the range of milligrams, while in the case of a drug in which the average dose is a gram or thereabouts, the toxic dose is likely to be in the range of several grams. In this relative sense, a drug prescribed in milligrams is no safer than one prescribed in grams, and potency in terms of absolute weight is important only in measuring out the dose. As already pointed out, the danger in drugs exists in the relationship between toxic and therapeutic dose, and not in weight alone; as a corollary, safety exists only in terms of how many times the average dose may be exceeded without danger, namely in a wide therapeutic range.

Variations in Potency

Because many of our drugs are made synthetically and controlled in manufacture, they are usually of constant composition and potency. Variations in potency occur, however, in many drugs which are still obtained from plants. The amount of a particular drug in a plant depends on a number of things: the variety or strain of the plant, fertilization of the soil, weather conditions during the growing season, method of storage and degree to which the crude material has been purified. For these reasons the amount of drug in plant preparations varies considerably from year to year, from batch to batch and from one part of the world to another. When it is possible to extract pure crystalline material from plant preparations, as in the case of quinine, the medication is of uniform and constant purity, but this is not always the case with medication of plant or biologic origin.

Standards of Potency and Purity

In order to insure the constancy of drugs, standards of composition, potency and purity are set by federal law. Physicians have the assurance that what they prescribe remains the same regardless of the pharmacist from whom it is purchased, the part of the country in which it is bought, and the date of the filling of the prescription. This precaution is essential to the health of the nation and the efficient practice of medicine.

A committee of physicians, pharmacologists, pharmacists and drug manufacturers meets regularly to discuss drugs in common use, to devise standards and means of testing for composition and to change old regulations to conform with advances in medical knowledge and practice. This committee advises the United States Congress of its decisions and every ten years an official and legal compilation of important drugs, their composition, and tests for their purity and potency is published. This is known as the *United States Pharmacopeia*, usually called U.S.P., and designated by the number of its edition. The latest is U.S.P. XIV and was published in

1950. This is a legal document as well as a reference book, and it contains legal standards for the official drugs used throughout this country and its possessions. Drugs listed therein are given official names, such as Digitoxin, U.S.P.

The U.S.P., however, does not list all drugs and drug mixtures still in use; only those are included which the committee considers important enough and well enough established to list. Thus many of the older drugs which are still used by older practitioners have been excluded from recent editions of the U.S.P. Some of these may be found in the *National Formulary* (N.F.) which sets legal standards for the drugs and mixtures which it lists and which includes older drugs no longer in the U.S.P. Neither U.S.P. nor N.F. contain trade names or extremely new and untried drugs.

Still another listing is published by the American Medical Association. This is an annual volume called *New and Nonofficial Remedies* (N.N.R.) which lists and describes many drugs manufactured under patents and copyrights, owned by manufacturers and usually not under the control of U.S.P. regulations. Drugs listed and described in N.N.R. have passed a review board of the American Medical Association; acceptance for N.N.R. implies that the drug is useful and that the claims for it are founded on substantial evidence and are not excessive.

There are many drugs not to be found in any of the official or nonofficial books just described. They may have been omitted because they are archaic, useless, too toxic, or sometimes in the case of a useful trade-named drug, unethically advertised. These may be found in many scattered sources, the largest of which is the Dispensatory. These are published privately and entirely unofficially; they list and describe drugs and mixtures of drugs of all types and varieties without reference to usefulness. Yet in spite of this, there are so many drugs, and so many different names for the same drugs, that it is occasionally impossible to find an official reference to some of them. Consider, for example, the fact that one trade publication lists about 850 different vitamin preparations alone.

Drug Assay

The potency of drug preparations must be determined by some means if they are to be kept constant. Natural variations may exceed

300 per cent in the case of some drugs obtained from different batches of the same plant. There is also the fact that some drug manufacturers may be tempted to adulterate or mislabel drugs for profit. In order to insure a properly labeled product and that the unethical as well as the ethical drug manufacturers mean the same thing when they indicate the content of a tablet or capsule on a label, drugs are constantly being tested by the Pure Food and Drug Division of the United States Department of Agriculture. The better drug manufacturers do a great deal of drug testing on their own before they package drugs.

Assaying or testing of drugs may be performed chemically or biologically. In many instances it is possible to determine the amount of a particular drug present in a preparation by chemical test. This is the simplest and the most certain way of determining the potency and purity of drugs.

In some cases, it is not technically possible to determine the amount of a drug present by chemical test, and the biologic method must be used. This is known as *bio-assay*. Since bio-assay is rarely needed for synthetic drugs, it is mainly used for those of plant or animal origin which cannot be completely purified or crystallized. In bio-assay the amount of drug necessary to produce a particular pharmacologic effect on an animal (hence biologic testing) is determined. Thus in the case of epinephrine, the ability of a preparation to raise a dog's blood pressure is determined; in the case of digitalis leaf the effect on a cat's heart is determined, while in the case of extract of the posterior pituitary gland, the effect on the uterus of a guinea-pig is tested. In the case of each drug, the amount necessary to produce a specific effect of this type is designated as a unit. Thus there is a unit of digitalis and a unit of posterior pituitary extract. A strong, active, specimen of the drug in question is usually selected as a standard material and the amount of this material necessary to produce an effect of one unit is determined. When this is done by the Pharmacopoeial committee, the material is known as a U.S.P. Reference Standard, and the unit, a U.S.P. unit.

When a specimen of a drug is to be tested, it is compared with the U.S.P. Reference Standard in the test animal. If it is stronger, less of this material than the standard is necessary to provide one unit of drug, and conversely, if it is weaker, more of the specimen than of the standard is required for one unit of drug. The drug may be so labeled, or it can be altered in composition by mixing with stronger or weaker specimens until the mixture conforms with U.S.P. standard potency. It should be clear that a unit may not be a weighable amount of a drug, but an amount which produces a particular biologic effect on a test animal.

The Patient and the Dose

The amount of a particular drug which will produce a specific effect varies with patients; one may be more sensitive and another less sensitive to the same material. Sometimes individual variations are rather wide and one patient may require three times as much as another to produce identical effects. There is no way of determining in advance and without trial where a particular patient will fall in the range of dosage. In some cases one may find that it is not at all possible to duplicate in one patient what may be produced with ease in another.

Age and Weight

But factors other than individual sensitivity enter into drug response. The age and weight of a patient play a role. Obviously an infant would require much less of a drug than a full-grown adult. Within limits this relationship between size or weight and dosage is important; in general it applies to the large categories, namely, infants, children, adults. More accurate applications of dose to size are not usually necessary. There are a few exceptions, however, in which weight-dosage relationship seems to be especially important, and in such cases patients are weighed before dosage is estimated.

There are several formulas for dosage in infants, none of which is infallible. One system uses a weight relationship, taking the average adult to weigh 50 kilograms. The infant's or child's weight, divided by this, is then used to determine the fraction of the average adult dose which will be used. Still another formula is Cowling's rule. The age of the child at his next birthday is divided by 24, with the resulting fraction equal to the fraction of the adult dose to be used. Young's rule also uses age to determine the fraction of the adult dose. This is arrived at by taking the child's age and dividing it by 12 plus the age.

Sex

Another factor which plays a role in drug response is the sex of the patient. Obviously, in the case of the sex hormones, different responses are obtained from the same materials in each sex.

Disease

The disease of the patient may also play a role in determining drug response, and hence the dosage which may be applied. Some diseases require higher dosage of drugs than are needed for the same effects in health, and some diseases require more drug than other diseases. Thus in subacute bacterial endocarditis, far larger doses of penicillin are needed than for almost any other disease which responds to penicillin treatment. In some instances the disease may interfere with the absorption or the elimination of the drug. If a drug is eliminated by the kidneys it may not be normally eliminated by a patient with serious kidney disease. In such a case only a smaller than average dose might be safe. If disease prevents or intereferes with absorption, far larger doses than ordinarily used might be necessary.

Individual Idiosyncracies

Due to special sensitivities many patients may be able to accept only very small doses without discomforts of one sort or another. These may assume a variety of forms. In some cases patients suffer from the usual minor toxic symptoms, or even major toxic symptoms from unusually small doses; in other instances they develop symptoms not usually seen with the drug, such as unusual forms of gastrointestinal disturbances, fevers, rashes, joint pains, bleeding gums, blood dyscrasias, etc. Some patients have found in their own experience, either through self-medication or with the guidance of a physician, that they are susceptible to particular drugs and have good results from others. Many people, for example, have their favorite cathartic, which they have found works better for them, or causes less distress, than others.

Such differences in response are also found in analgesics, hypnotics, and other potent drugs with which the patient has had experience. A number of patients, for example, vomit violently from an injection of morphine. This would be a serious reaction in the case of a patient who is suffering from an acute heart attack. If the patient has previously had a vomiting reaction from a drug and so informs the nurse, she should promptly relay this information to the doctor.

Psychologic considerations may play an important role in these judgments of patients. Nevertheless, there is no reason to ignore them completely, for sometimes they may be the only warnings which will prevent a disaster. When there is no reason for not heeding the patient, his choice should be given serious consideration, for even if there is a strong psychologic element in these patient choices, there is no good reason for not taking advantage of the part psychic factors play in curing disease.

Route of Administration

The route of administration also affects dosage. In general, the most effective route is intravenous as it usually requires a smaller dose to produce the same effects as the same drug given by other routes. This is so because the drug reaches its peak concentration in the bloodstream very quickly and without loss of drug through incomplete absorption, rapid elimination, or destruction. Other parenteral routes, the intramuscular and subcutaneous, usually require more drug to produce effects of the same intensity. When given by the oral route, most drugs require several times as much material as when given by vein.

It is well to remember, however, that there are important exceptions to this rule. In the case of digitoxin, for example, the dose of the drug by mouth and by vein is identical. This is so because the drug is completely absorbed from the gastro-intestinal tract and is very slowly eliminated. Absorption and elimination are the factors which determine the relative size of parenteral and oral doses.

Duration of Effects

Another important consideration in determining dosage is duration of effects. In some cases a single dose produces all the effect that is desired. For example, in the relief of the painful spasm of the coronary artery in angina pectoris, the patient gets his relief from a single dose of nitroglycerin and takes no more until he again experiences pain. Prolonged effects are needed when the condition under treatment is one which persists. Here a continued level of drug action is usually required. In the case of a patient who needs digitalis over a period of years, a single dose may be taken every day to maintain the effect. This is an adequate dosage because the drug is slowly absorbed and eliminated. In the case of an infection treated with penicillin, one now has a choice between the administration of intramuscular doses of penicillin every 3 or 4 hours in order to maintain the effect "round-the-clock," or giving doses of so-called "depot" penicillin every 24 to 48 hours which is slowly absorbed and produces prolonged effects. In the latter case the single dose would be many times the single dose given repeatedly by intramuscular injection, for it would have to serve 24 to 48 hours, instead of 3 to 4 hours.

Maintenance Dosage

Maintenance dosage, often distinguished from initial dosage, is a self-explanatory term: it refers to the dosage of drugs necessary to maintain an effect which has already been established. How long this effect should or can be safely maintained depends on the nature of the drug and the disease being treated. The schedule necessary for maintenance has already been indicated. It depends on the rate at which the drug is eliminated or destroyed in the body; the more rapidly the drug disappears, for whatever reason, the more frequently doses have to be given.

In order to simplify the nursing problems in the maintenance of drug effects for those which are relatively rapidly eliminated, devices are sometimes possible which store the drug in the body in a form which permits small amounts to be absorbed continuously over an extended period of time. The best known of these devices is the repository or depot form of penicillin in which a dose of the slowly absorbed form of penicillin, enough to last for from 24 to 72 hours, is injected intramuscularly at one time. In the muscle this form of penicillin forms a depot which supplies the drug to the body for from one to three days, depending on the form of penicillin and the total dose injected. This eliminates the need for injections every three or four hours. Obviously the dose for depot effects must be far larger than each single repeated dose of the rapidly absorbed form of penicillin.

Average Dose

A drug's average dose is usually stated in definite terms in texts on pharmacology and reference books on drugs, as if it had an absolute meaning. This expression, average dose, often is not well understood. When it is applied without understanding, the use of drugs may become ineffectual or dangerous, or both.

The average dose is a figure arrived at by a mathematical trick, which considers safety first, effective results second and the average person in the population last. It may be defined as a dose of a drug which will produce a therapeutic effect in a significant proportion of the population while producing toxic effects in a few. In most instances, therefore, it is more likely to be safe than effective. The average dose may also be well described as the safe "starting" dose.

This discussion about the average dose arises from the fact that the reactions of humans to drugs is just about as different as their faces; as already explained, doses which are ineffectual for some are toxic for others, and there is no way of telling in advance of actual experience with the particular drug in the particular patient under the circumstances that exist at the moment of administration. This is the situation that calls for art in the administration of drugs. The average dose, therefore, is one which may safely be used in most cases to start the therapeutic experiment and to find out more precisely how the drug is subsequently to be used in the patient. What the final schedule of dosage may be, depends largely on the therapeutic and toxic reactions the patient may experience from the "average" or safe "starting" dose. As has been pointed out, toxicity as well as therapeutic effect, plays an important role in determining the average dose.

Toxicity

The dose of the drug must not be so large as to harm or endanger the patient. If a drug has a high therapeutic index, the average dose can safely be one which will be effective in a relatively large proportion of patients. In the case of a drug with a low therapeutic index, namely one in which the therapeutic and the toxic doses are not far apart, the average dose, for reasons of safety, is likely to be below the therapeutic level in a large proportion of cases.

Determining Dosage

In summary the best working dosage is determined by experiment in each case, the outcome depending on several unpredictables: (1) the patient's sensitivity to toxic properties of the drug, (2) the sensitivity of the patient or his disease to the therapeutic effects of the drug and (3) the circumstances which determine how the drug should best be applied in the particular case. The average dose, as described in texts, is not necessarily the dose which the average patient may find therapeutically effective and safe; it is merely the dose which is not likely to cause serious toxic reactions and may, in addition, induce useful therapeutic actions. The final dose for the patient is one tailored to fit him, his disease, and the circumstances and may frequently differ radically from the average dose stated in textbooks.

Study Questions

1. Where, in the United States, may we find legal standards of composition, purity and potency of drugs?
2. Where may we find official names of drugs?
3. How is drug potency determined?
4. What factors modify dosage of drugs?

5

ADMINISTRATION OF DRUGS

The way in which a drug may best be administered depends on many factors: (1) whether a local or a systemic effect is needed, (2) whether the patient is conscious, (3) whether the patient is vomiting, (4) the characteristics of the drug itself which determine whether it may be given orally or must be given parenterally, (5) the safety of parenteral administration, (6) whether an emergency demands the most rapid method of obtaining effects regardless of dangers, (7) frequency of dosage.

Forms of Administration

Other less pressing matters also enter into a decision of the exact means of administration, as for example, the amount of drug to be given at one time. In the case of a drug to be given in very large amounts, small pills or capsules would make it a tedious matter, and for that matter patients tend to resent or resist taking a great many pills at one time. Bitter drugs are best given in a form which either masks the taste or prevents tasting, such as a capsule. If the patient is a child, a flavoring material should be chosen which is acceptable to a child. Some drugs are easier to take by mouth when they are cold. Some drugs have persistent bad taste, and this can sometimes be shortened by following the dose with a cold drink, ginger ale or perhaps orange juice. These are all devices which the nurse should learn, which not only make matters more pleasant for the patient, but also insure cooperation, thus making matters simpler for the nurse.

The frequency of dosage is sometimes a very important practical matter in determining the means of administration. When a drug

has to be given every few hours round-the-clock, the patient is
soon apt to develop a resistance to taking the drug, especially if the
mode of administration is unpleasant. A patient will often take the
most unpleasant material once or twice, but not willingly do so at
frequent intervals. In the case of drugs given by injection, frequent
dosage is apt to set up a firm resentment not only against the medication, but also possibly against the nurse and the doctor.

Medications are often colored for psychologic reasons and patients tend to identify them by color, even though it may be due to
a dye rather than to the drug itself. This sometimes complicates
matters, for the same prescription made up by another pharmacist
may look a little different from the first preparation because of a
variation in the tint used. It is sometimes difficult to explain satisfactorily to the patient that this difference in appearance does not
mean an essential difference in the medication.

Often a patient will ask a nurse to identify a medication by its
color. When there are established color codes for capsules the nurse
will add to her authority by acquainting herself with the codes. On
the other hand, identification by color is not always possible, especially with solutions and the so-called extemporaneous prescription.

Mixtures

Mixtures of drugs would at first glance seem to be a way of simplifying the burden of administering medications. This simplification
is more apparent than real, even in the case of drugs which may
safely be mixed together. Sometimes mixtures may be the cause of
serious difficulties, and in general, the modern tendency is to use
them as little as possible and to prescribe drugs in the simplest
practical preparation.

Since few drugs are excreted from the body at exactly the same
rate, in a mixture of active drugs, each may be excreted at a different rate. In a situation in which more of the effect of one drug of a
mixture is required more of all the accompanying drugs, whether
needed or not, are also given at the same time. If these drugs are
more slowly excreted or are more toxic than the first, repetition of
doses, in order to obtain a more intense effect with one drug in
the mixture, may result in undesirably intense effects and even

serious toxic effects due to the others. There is also the fact that each additional drug in a mixture increases the possibility of an allergic reaction. For these reasons many physicians follow the principle of giving the simplest possible prescription at all times, and using mixtures only when it clearly serves a useful purpose.

A common practice in older medicine was to give extremely complicated prescriptions consisting of many drugs, sometimes ten or more. In the vast majority of cases this practice was the result of both ignorance and a dearth of useful and effective drugs. The complicated or so-called shot-gun prescription was given in the hope that one of its many ingredients might do some good. This practice has tended to disappear with the development of modern medicine and effective therapeutics.

Measurement of Medication

No matter how accurate the diagnosis, how carefully therapy is planned, or how sympathetically the nurse administers the medication, it all will have been useless if the dosage is not precisely measured—if the patient is to benefit and not to be hurt by treatment. It is well to remember that if too little medicine is given no good will come of it; if too much, the patient may die. The person who measures the medicine is in a crucial position in the final test of the therapy. The careless nurse can here undo all the good of medicine.

Usually it is a relatively simple thing to measure out the dose of a drug, especially in these times, as so many drugs are already made up in fixed forms, tablets, capsules, ampules and the like. There are still many instances, however, in which the nurse must measure the medication rather than simply counting pills. Therefore, she must understand the weights and measures used in medicine. If she fails to do this her ministrations might be more dangerous than useful.

At the present time, two systems of weights and measures are in use: the Apothecary and the Metric Systems. The former is the older system; it is used only in English-speaking countries and is rightfully dying out. The latter is simpler, more scientific and easier. It is used throughout the continent of Europe, and is rapidly coming into use in modern hospitals in this country. It is the system used in this book. But since both systems are still widely used in this country, nursing students must not only learn both, but learn how to translate one into the other with reasonable facility. The details of these matters are fully discussed in Part III, The Medicine.

Study Questions

1. What factors influence the methods of administration of drugs?
2. Why are mixtures of drugs frequently contraindicated?
3. What do we mean by the term "fixed forms"? Give examples.

6

PREPARATION OF DRUGS AND MEDICAMENTS

Source

One of the ways in which drugs are classified is according to their source: (1) plants, (2) minerals, (3) micro-organisms, (4) insects, (5) animals, (6) air, (7) synthetic. The first drugs were obtained from plants but modern chemistry has made it possible to reproduce many of them synthetically in the laboratory. In addition, many new drugs, never before known nor found anywhere in nature, have come from the synthetic chemist's laboratory.

In drugs of plant origin, the entire plant may be used, but usually only a part of it is used; in some cases the root, the leaf, the stem, the flower, the bark, or the seed is the most effective in medicinal content. For example, digitalis comes from the leaf, morphine from the flower and quinine from the bark of the plants of their origin.

Active Principles

Active principles are the ingredients of the plant which give it its pharmacologic properties. The unrefined plants or the simple extracts are mixtures of many substances, most of which are pharmacologically inert, some of which may be irritant and usually only a very small proportion of which is the active principle. In most instances the crude mixture can be used just as effectively as the purified active principle, providing that a large enough dose is given to compensate for the large amount of incidental material present. In some cases, however, the impurities may be undesirable, and all or nearly all of the nonmedicinal materials must be removed before the preparation can safely be used as a medicament.

Types of Drugs

A few of the common groups of drugs, classified according to their source and chemical nature are defined below.

Alkaloids are a large group of active principles of vegetable origin (or made synthetically) with an alkaline reaction, usually highly insoluble in water but soluble in acids, with an intensely bitter taste, usually effective in very small doses. Morphine, caffeine, quinine, nicotine, atropine and strychnine are among the best known alkaloids.

Antibiotics are elaborated by micro-organisms in their normal life processes and inhibit or destroy other micro-organisms. These materials are extracted from the media on which the micro-organisms grow. Outstanding examples are penicillin, streptomycin, tetracycline, erythromycin, bacitracin.

Antitoxins are concentrated extracts of animal serum containing specific antibodies which neutralize bacterial toxins but do not affect the bacteria themselves. Diphtheria and tetanus antitoxins are examples.

Chemotherapeutic agents are chemicals, as contrasted with biologic agents such as antitoxins and antibiotics, which are usually made synthetically. Well known chemotherapeutic agents are the sulfonamide drugs and salvarsan for syphilis.

Enzymes are living ferments which are capable of producing changes only when they are alive. The best known enzymes are those involved in the digestive processes, such as pepsin.

Glycosides (*or glucosides*) form a large group of active principles of plant origin (not yet made synthetically) which contain a sugar fraction in a complex molecule. The best known glycosides are the digitalis drugs.

Hormones are materials normally elaborated in the animal body, which exert an effect on distant parts of the body. Hormones may be obtained by extraction from organs of cattle or other animals or made synthetically. Cortisone, insulin and thyroid extract are examples.

Serums are blood concentrates which contain specific curative antibodies. They are obtained from humans or animals who have had the disease and survived. An example is meningococcus serum.

Vaccines are living, attenuated or dead bacteria or viruses which are used to induce an active immunity against a disease, hence, mainly as prophylactic agents. Vaccine virus is used against smallpox, typhoid vaccine against typhoid fever.

Physical and Chemical Properties

Physical and chemical properties of drugs vary greatly. Some drugs are light and fluffy, some heavy, some bitter, some sweet, some liquid, some solid, some gaseous, some crystalline, some amorphous, some soluble, some insoluble, some are acid, some are alkaline, some deteriorate rapidly, some last forever without change, some react chemically with other drugs, some are relatively inert chemically. These are matters of practical importance because they determine (1) the means by which drugs may be extracted and purified, (2) how they may be administered, (3) to some degree, the rate of absorption and elimination, (4) whether they may be mixed with other drugs, (5) how they should be stored.

The methods used for the extraction and purification are obviously determined by the chemical nature of the drugs and their solubility in the various extraction materials. Drugs can be administered in solution only if they are dissolved in a solvent which may be safely injected or taken by mouth. There have been many disasters from toxic solvents used in preparations containing entirely safe drugs.

Highly insoluble materials tend to be more slowly absorbed than the more soluble ones, although this is not always the case and there are highly soluble drugs which are poorly absorbed and insoluble drugs which are well absorbed. If drugs react with each other chemically, there is usually sufficient alteration in pharmacologic properties to make the mixture useless. For this reason physically and chemically reactive drugs are considered incompatible and are not mixed in the same solution, although they may be taken by mouth if only a short interval separates their administration.

Many drugs are available in different chemical forms or salts. Thus there is morphine and morphine sulfate, codeine, codeine sulfate and codeine phosphate, sulfadiazine and sodium sulfadiazine. In the vast majority of cases there is no difference in the pharmacologic effects of the parent substance and its salts. In the main the differences are matters of solubility, taste, and rarely absorption.

In general, alkaloids, such as morphine and codeine, are highly insoluble while their salts are very soluble. The parent form of the sulfonamide drugs is relatively insoluble while the sodium salt is very soluble. In all these cases, the soluble form of the drug must be used when the drug is to be administered by the injection of a solution, but when the same drug is to be given by mouth, it is a matter of indifference which form is used.

It is not to be assumed that solubility in a salt of a drug provides advantages in absorption; this is only sometimes true. In most cases it is interesting to note that the acid of the stomach and the alkali of the intestine convert drugs into the same form regardless of the particular salt or form administered by mouth. The same is largely true in the case of the action of the chemical elements of the tissues and the blood on drugs which are administered by the parenteral route.

Because there is no difference in the pharmacologic nature of the various forms of the same drug they will not be distinguished and, in general, the salts will not be mentioned. It will be pointed out, however, when a particular form of a drug has special significance.

Deterioration

Deterioration is an important characteristic of many drugs, especially those of biologic origin. This is a property which varies with each drug.

Certain physical forces tend to accelerate drug deterioration. Solutions, in general, deteriorate more rapidly than dry preparations. Acid or alkalai may accelerate deterioration. Direct exposure to sunlight, heat, the presence of oxygen or air and the presence of impurities may also accelerate drug deterioration. For these reasons many drugs will keep much longer in the dry and pure form, in a well filled and well stoppered bottle, away from the direct sunlight, or in a refrigerator. Which of these precautions is important varies; in some cases all are necessary, in some none.

There are instances in which the products of deterioration may be harmful. In all instances deterioration reduces the potency of the drug so that it may no longer correspond with the label. Precautions which are essential are indicated in the Materia Medica in this book. Some solutions change color on standing; this is often, but not always a sign of significant deterioration. When one is uncertain, it is safest to discard discolored solutions of medication, especially in the case of a parenteral preparation. Thus, it becomes important for the nurse to know the normal color of a preparation.

It is also important in each case to examine the package for instructions on storage and an expiration date. If the storage precautions have not been followed, or the expiration date has been passed, the preparation should not be used.

Pharmaceutical Preparations

Drugs used for pharmacologic effects have to be put into a form that is possible to administer. Drugs that have to be applied on the skin must be made up in a suitable form. Drugs that are to be put up in fluid form not only have to be dissolved, but they have to remain in solution; if they are to be emulsified, the proper emulsifying agent must be used. If the patient refuses to take his medication regularly the best laid therapeutic plans will fail. This involves other problems in preparation, as some drugs are so bitter they are impossible to take, and others are so irritant that taking them may injure the mouth.

Taste is an important consideration when drugs are given orally. For this reason the nurse should acquaint herself with the taste of the medications with which she deals, and learn how best to disguise it. The flavoring materials used in drugs have no influence on drug action itself, but the fact that they enable the patient to take the drug is an exceedingly important feature. The taste of drugs is an important medical and nursing problem, in adults as well as in children.

Drugs may be prepared in such fixed forms as tablets, pills, capsules, powders, etc. These have the advantage of accuracy in dose measurement. Although the problem of taste is avoided with capsules and coated tablets some patients have difficulty in swallowing them and will refuse to take them.

Fluid medications are sometimes colored. This is usually done for psychologic reasons and is sometimes especially important for the actual color of the mixture may be such as to suggest deterioration to the patient.

The pharmacist uses many materials in his attempt to make acceptable and professional-appearing preparations. Among the groups of substances he uses the following may be listed: antioxidants, binders, emulsifiers, flavors, colors, preservatives, solvents, stabilizers, bases, ointments, vehicles.

In some instances pills, capsules and other fixed forms are

colored. These colors sometimes represent a code, for example, pentobarbital sodium is usually placed in a yellow capsule, the 0.2 mg. tablet of digitoxin is usually white, while the 0.1 mg. tablet of the same drug is usually pink. Although the nurse should learn these codes, she should not rely on color when administering medicine to patients.

Pharmaceuticals

There is a large variety of pharmaceutic preperations which are used to facilitate the administration and application of drugs. The more commonly used ones are listed and described below.

Aromatic waters are aqueous solutions of volatile oils. They are used as flavoring vehicles for water-soluble drugs.

Cachets are wafers of starch or flour which enclose a drug much in the same way as a capsule. They are readily soluble or may be swallowed whole.

Capsules are gelatin containers and may be swallowed without tasting the drug contained. The hard capsule is used for dry materials, the soft capsule for oils, oleoresins and solutions of drugs in oils.

Cerates are preparations which contain wax to prevent them from melting at body temperature.

Collodions are solutions of active drugs in collodion, ether and alcohol which are used for external application only.

Confections or electuaries are candy-like preparations of drugs.

Decoctions are aqueous preparations of vegetable drugs which contain about 5 per cent of the drug.

Effervescent salts are mixtures which bubble when mixed with water.

Elixirs are cordial-like drug preparations which contain alcohol, sugar and aromatic flavors.

Emulsions are aqueous preparations of drugs which will not dissolve and are suspended in a vehicle by means of an emulsifying agent.

Enemata are liquid preparations for rectal administration.

Extracts are concentrated extracts of drugs made by dissolving out the active materials and concentrating the extract by evaporation.

Fluid extracts are liquid extracts of drugs of such strength that each cubic centimeter represents 1 gram of the original material.

Glycerites are solutions of drugs in glycerin.

Infusions are aqueous extracts of vegetable drugs which generally represent 5 per cent of the original material.

Lamella are small discs containing drug to be applied directly to the eyeball.

Liniments are alcohol, soap or oil preparations of drugs generally applied externally with rubbing.

Lotions are aqueous liquid preparations for local application.

Masses are soft, solid preparations which are usually made into pills.

Mixtures are combinations of more than one drug with a fluid vehicle, which may form a clear solution, an emulsion, or an unstable suspension.

Mucilages are aqueous solutions of gummy materials.

Oils. Fixed oils are the normal neutral fats or oils of plant or animal origin, such as are commonly found in foodstuffs. *Volatile* or *essential oils* are usually aromatic or tasty, highly fluid oils obtained from plants, often used for flavoring or giving aroma to medicaments.

Ointments are soft, greasy preparations for spreading on the skin.

Oleoresins are thick liquid preparations obtained by extraction from vegetable drugs containing resins and volatile oils.

Papers are dry powdered drugs in which each individual dose is folded into a paper which is opened before use.

Pastes are ointment-like preparations of drugs in a nonfatty base for application to the skin.

Pills are spherical or globular bits of medication which may be swallowed easily.

Plasters are solid preparations for external use.

Poultices are soft, solid preparations to produce heat in a localized area of the body by external application.

Powders are medications administered in the dry powdered form, often in a paper.

Solutions are preparations in which the drug is completely dissolved in a liquid vehicle.

Spirits are alcoholic solutions.

Suppositories are solid preparations for introduction into the rectum or vagina to produce local or systemic effects.

Sirups are solutions of drugs in sirup.

Tablets. Compressed tablets are hard discs of medicament and vehicle for oral administration. In order to prevent passage through the intestine without solution, the tablets often contain a material which makes them break up into small fragments when they reach the stomach or small intestine. *Tablets triturate* are small fragile tablets made by moulding without pressure, which break up very easily. *Enteric-coated tablets* have a coating which is impervious to the acid of the stomach so that the active drug passes untouched to the intestine. This is done either to prevent destruction of the drug by the gastric juices or to protect the stomach from irritation in cases in which the stomach is sensitive to the particular drug.

Tinctures are hydro-alcoholic extracts or solutions of drugs, which usually represent about 10 Gm. of drug for each 100 cc. of tincture.

Troches or lozenges are flat discs containing drug to be dissolved slowly in the mouth to produce an effect on the mucous membrane of the mouth or throat.

In addition to this rather long list of preparations, the manufacturers of drugs are constantly introducing their own preparations and providing them with still other names. This is done in order to identify the product as their own and to encourage the purchase of their specific brand. On the market at this writing, for example, are such forms as "Dosules" and "Spansules," definitions for which cannot be found in any standard medical reference. Thus the drug manufacturer helps to confuse the issue by giving odd and meaningless names to physical forms of preparations as well as to the drugs themselves.

Study Questions

1. Indicate some disadvantages and advantages of crude forms of drugs.

2. In what ways do the chemical and physical properties of drugs effect their administration and use?

3. What are some of the practical points for the nurse to consider in the administration of drugs to patients?

4. What is the purpose of enteric coated medications?

7

AN APPROACH TO DRUGS

The nurse should establish a general attitude to drugs, a way of thinking, examining and using them—old ones as well as new ones. The nurse is, of course, not often the one who chooses the drug to use, but since she is constantly with the patient, she is in the best position to see what good it is doing and what its undesirable effects may be. What should the nurse do in the case of a new drug? What should she find out about the drugs she handles? What are the facts which are essential to the understanding and meaningful handling of drugs? Here are some questions the nurse should be able to answer:

1. What are the therapeutic actions and indications for the drug?
2. What are the contraindications?
3. How well is it absorbed from the gastro-intestinal tract?
4. What are the permissible routes of administration?
5. How quickly do effects develop by each route?
6. How is it eliminated?
7. How long does complete elimination take?
8. What is the average dose?
9. How often should doses be given?
10. What are the minor and major toxic symptoms?
11. How is toxicity treated?
12. In the case of intolerance, what drug may be substituted?
13. Does the drug deteriorate?
14. How should it be stored?

At first glance this seems like an impressive list of questions, but many of the items can be compressed, and one soon learns to find out all of these things about a drug automatically. These questions are answered for most of the drugs listed in the Materia Medica of this book. In some cases all of the information is contained in a very short paragraph, yet despite its brevity the nurse will gain a comprehension of the drugs she handles. Such an understanding will not only bring positive advantages in the therapeutic effects of drugs but it will also reduce the incidence of serious toxic reactions. The nurse will recognize the untoward effects in their earliest stages and apply the proper measures before there is further intensification of the poisoning.

Misuse of Drugs

Serious dangers may come from the misuse of drugs. They must never be given indiscriminately or sloppily applied; both the mental and the mechanical processes involved in their administration must be careful and precise. When it is decided to treat a patient, the program for treatment must be effective, carefully planned and skillfully executed. Dosage and measurement must be accurate. Serious losses to the patient, the community, the practice of medicine and the art of nursing will come from less.

If the dose is too small it may fail to cure or to help the patient; if it is too large it may poison or kill the patient. In the case of a new drug, misuse and the poor results which inevitably follow may damage its reputation and discourage its proper use in cases which would benefit from it. A single poor result tends to prejudice one against the further use of a drug.

The use of sub-therapeutic doses of effective chemotherapeutic or antibiotic drugs may enable bacteria to develop a resistance to the drugs to the degree that it is later impossible to treat the infection with any safe dose. Such drug resistance, once developed, is transmitted by bacteria to their progeny. Thus it is within the realm of possibility that such poor use of drugs will result in a widespread drug-resistant form of the disease. Diseases may cease to yield to our "miracle" drugs. This is not a purely theoretical worry. It seems already to have happened in the case of gonorrhea and the sulfonamide drugs which once were used so successfully to treat it. Fortunately in this instance, penicillin still remains an effective cure for gonorrhea. So great is the fear in some quarters for this kind of loss of therapeutic potential, that in the case of the new anti-tuberculosis drug, isonicotinic acid hydrazide, a warning has been issued to all physicians to use the drug with the greatest consideration for indications and adequate dosage.

The use of drugs in conditions not requiring them or unresponsive to them, may stimulate an allergy to the drug in the patient. At some other time, when his life or his health depends on it, the patient may not be able to take the drug.

The medical and the nursing professions have had a serious responsibility placed in their hands in recent years. In addition to taking care of the health and lives of patients, we have also had to accept the responsibility for the preservation of the effectiveness of our "miracle" drugs. We must guard these new and valuable tools with all the care and consideration which they require and deserve —or we may lose them.

Approach to New Drugs

In the last twenty years the treatment of infectious disease has been revolutionized by some new drugs, but this is only one side of the picture. Most of us seem to forget that there have also been new drugs which have been disappointing, and others which have even proved harmful. There are grave dangers in new and untested drugs, yet unless they are tried out, the new cures which can result from them will never be established. Those who practice medicine must be cautious on the one hand, but willing to try on the other.

One finds a few physicians and nurses who take a firm and obstructive attitude to new drugs. They disparage research and flatly state that, despite all evidence to the contrary, medical research has yielded little of fundamental importance. A careless attitude in the other direction is equally obstructive to progress. For there are some, in their great desire to find cures for as yet incurable disease, who are enthusiastic and indiscriminate about all drugs whose claims—still lacking in evidence—are in a desireable direction. These enthusiasts use no critical thinking about new drugs, and as a result they and their patients soon fall victim to false hopes and bad results. But there are some in medicine who have a healthy attitude to new drugs, who recognize the need for them, who know how to examine them and the reports made about them and, finally, who know how to evaluate the results they see in their own patients. This is an attitude which permits both caution and trial, and which favors progress.

In deciding on the value of all drugs, new and old, it is important to bear in mind the potent psychic elements which enter into the patient's reaction to his disease and the bias of the physician and the nurse. Everyone concerned in the treatment of a patient is so anxious for a cure that all tend to see the brighter side of the picture. Patients, nurses, doctors, relatives, all want the patient to feel and look better. They are most anxious that the medication they are using should be effective, and if they are attempting a therapeutic experiment with a new drug, they are anxious for the drug to work. If it happens to be an incurable disease, no one is willing to see the drug fail, and every change in the patient—no matter how small or uncertain—is wishfully thought to be for the better and considered a beneficial action of the drug.

In addition, there is the force of publicity. Newspaper reporters always find a successful drug more newsworthy than a questionable or unsuccessful one, and a positive statement more attractive than a hesitant one. For this reason doubts are rarely stated in newspaper reports on new drugs; they all tend to be overenthusiastic. For these obvious reasons errors in judgments on new drugs are virtually always in the direction of its usefulness. A purely scientific and unemotional attitude is difficult to maintain in the face of all these pressures.

Overenthusiasm for useless drugs is not a harmless pastime; it always has unhappy effects. The more serious, the more devastating the disease for which the new cure is claimed, the more unpleasant the aftereffects of the fallible drugs. People with incurable diseases are, understandably, continuously searching for cures, and, as a consequence, they are easy prey not only for deluded but honest physicans who think they have a cure, but for outright fakers as well. Whenever a cure for an incurable disease is prematurely (i.e. without satisfactory testing) announced, hordes of incurables make pilgrimages to the city from which the reports have come. To make this trip, many sell their homes or borrow money. Often they come in great numbers to small cities which are unable, medically or otherwise, to accommodate the sick and the dying. And when the cure fails, hundreds or thousands are stranded and without hope, depending on charity for shelter, food and fare home, or if they die, for burial. The tragic results of unfounded "cures" should not be forgotten when spreading information that a new drug, especially an untested one, seems to be the solution for an as yet incurable condition.

A common argument is, that for some reasons, the organized medical profession deliberately and maliciously keeps new cures in the dark. It is well to remember in this connection that no important drugs in recent years have been discovered by the newspaper profession. Such important drugs as insulin, liver extract, sulfonamides, penicillin and other antibiotics, serums and vaccines, new cardiac drugs, cortisone, the new anti-tubercular drugs have all been discovered by members of organized medicine and the first reports have come through accredited medical journals, not newspapers. That the problem of cancer has not yet yielded to research is an unhappy fact, but it is not because there is a cure which the medical profession does not wish to disclose. It is well to point out that doctors have the same death rate from disease as the rest of the population; that there is no indication that medicine is keeping something for itself that it does not use freely for everyone else. And it is also well to remember that there are trial committees in all specialties of medicine which investigate any drug with important claims, providing its nature is not a secret, and it will be made freely available for public use if it proves effective.

The danger of toxicity of new drugs is one which can be relatively effectively controlled. The government no longer permits untried drugs to be sold, for many people have lost their lives from such untested "cures." Useful drugs may sometimes be toxic, but there is a clear justification for their use if the dangers of the disease outweigh the danger of the drugs. But it is just as clearly an immoral matter to use a useless drug and a criminal matter when it also happens to be a dangerous one. Recently strong safeguards have been set against the indiscriminate sale of untested drugs. All new drugs must be thoroughly tested, on man as well as on animals, before they can be put on sale. The examination consists of two parts: animal experiments which indicate the possible therapeutic uses and the toxic properties, and human experiments which are used to confirm and establish the final principles for its use by the medical profession. The animal experiments are performed in accredited laboratories, usually in medical colleges; the human experiments are conducted in hospitals under the supervision of trained observers. Every attempt is made in these investigations to eliminate bias in judgments, both by the patient and the physician. With sufficient experimental trial under well controlled conditions, the safety and potential values can be determined, and a routine of treatment by the general practitioner established. The drug is then made available for general use.

But this is not necessarily the end of the story, for sometimes the large-scale trial brings out difficulties or failures which the original tests and studies failed to indicate. These results determine whether the drug is more useful than others already in common use for the same conditions, whether it has advantages over older and accepted remedies, whether it will replace them or soon be discarded. While old and tried drugs have the advantages that come with experience, it is always a good thing to have another useful drug available.

It is important to bear in mind that despite all previous trial and experiment which established a drug, each administration to a patient is still another experiment, for each patient is different.

Study Questions

1. What knowledge should the nurse have about a specific drug before she administers it to a patient?

2. What factors should the nurse consider in relation to attitudes of patients, professional groups and the general public regarding new drugs?

8

DEFINITIONS

The effects of the application of drugs to cells, organs and pathogenic organisms, without reference to their usefulness in the treatment of disease are known as the pharmacologic actions. Often drugs are described in terms of pharmacologic actions, and a list of definitions of such actions follows. In addition, the end result of such actions may prove to be useful in the treatment of disease; these comprise the therapeutic actions of drugs, their practical application in disease. A list of definitions of therapeutic actions also follows.

Pharmacologic Classes of Drugs

Adrenergic drugs are autonomic drugs which produce effects similar to those of stimulation of the adrenal gland, and in general, to that of an injection of epinephrine. Also sympathomimetic drugs.

Adrenocortical hormones are hormonal drugs extracted from the cortex of the adrenal gland. There are many of these.

Adrenolytic drugs are autonomic drugs which antagonize the effects of stimulation of the adrenal gland, or of an injection of epinephrine. Also sympatholytic drugs.

Amino acid preparations are mixtures of amino acids usually prepared by the digestion of proteins.

Androgens are male sex hormones.

Antibiotics are drugs elaborated by micro-organisms and extracted from their growth media, which depress or destroy other micro-organisms in dilute solution.

Anticholinergic drugs are autonomic drugs which antagonize the effects of stimulation of the parasympathetic nervous system or of an injection of cholinergic drugs such as methacholine (mecholyl). Also vagolytic and parasympatholytic drugs.

Antihistaminic drugs are a large group of drugs which antagonize the effects of histamine and relieve allergic reactions.

51

Antimitotic drugs are those which depress the rate of mitosis or multiplication of cells. They are used in the treatment of cancer and allied conditions.

Antisympathomimetic drugs are autonomic drugs which antagonize the effects of stimulation of the sympathetic nervous system or of an injection of epinephrine. Also sympatholytic drugs.

Autonomic drugs are drugs which simulate the effects or antagonize the effects of stimulation of the autonomic nervous system. These may be divided into four groups of drugs: (1) adrenergic or sympathomimetic; (2) cholinergic, parasympathomimetic or vagomimetic; (3) sympatholytic or adrenolytic; (4) anticholinergic, vagolytic or parasympatholytic drugs.

Biologicals are drugs derived from animals.

Chemotherapeutic drugs are chemical agents which cure a disease.

Cholinergic drugs are autonomic drugs which simulate the effects of stimulation of the parasympathomimetic nervous system or of an injection of epinephrine. Also sympatholytic drugs.

Color and dyes are harmless and pharmacologically inert materials used to color medication.

Depressants are drugs which reduce cellular or organ activity or responsiveness.

Digitalis drugs comprise a large group of glycosidal materials derived from plants, not necessarily from digitalis plants, but with the same effects as digitalis on heart muscle.

Endocrine drugs are materials extracted from the endocrine glands of animals or their synthetic equivalents. *See* hormones.

Estrogens are female sex hormones.

Exchange resins are inert materials, which are not absorbed in the intestinal tract, but which have the property of combining tenaciously to particular ions (acid or alkali) in the intestinal tract.

Flavors are materials without pharmacologic action which are used to disguise the taste of medications.

Hormones are extracts of endocrine glands of animals or their synthetic equivalents. *See* endocrine drugs.

Narcotic drugs are a group of potent drugs which may induce coma. Some also present the special hazard of addiction, and for this reason they are carefully controlled by law.

Parasympatholytic drugs are autonomic drugs which antagonize the effects of stimulation of the parasympathetic nervous system or of an injection of methacholine. Also anticholinergic and vagolytic drugs.

Parasympathomimetic drugs are autonomic drugs which simulate the effects of stimulation of the parasympathetic nervous system or of cholinergic drugs such as methacholine. Also cholinergic drugs.

Parenteral fluids are fluids which may be injected parenterally, particularly intravenously, in large quantities in relative safety.

Pharmaceuticals are materials without pharmacologic actions which are used in the physical preparation of medications.

Solvents are pharmaceuticals which are used solely for their solvent actions.

Stimulants are drugs which increase cellular or organ activity or responsiveness.

Sympatholytic drugs are autonomic drugs which antagonize the effects of stimulation of the sympathetic nervous system or of an injection of epinephrine. Also adrenergic drugs.

Toxins are toxic products of bacterial activity.

Vaccines are attenuated or dead pathogenic micro-organisms.

Vagolytic drugs are autonomic drugs which antagonize the effects of stimulation of the parasympathetic nervous system or of an injection of methacholine. Also anticholinergic and parasympatholytic drugs.

Vitamins are essential food elements required only in minute amounts.

Therapeutic Classes of Drugs

Acidifiers are drugs which tend to induce an acid reaction.

Adsorbents are drugs which tend to combine with irritant materials by physical means.

Allergenic preparations are extracts of materials which may induce allergic reactions used either in testing or in desensitization.

Analeptics are drugs which induce convulsions and stimulate reflex activity.

Analgesics are drugs which tend to relieve pain. This term is usually applied to the nonhabit forming drugs.

Anesthetics are drugs which induce deep sleep or coma.

Antacids are drugs which combine with or neutralize acid, usually of the stomach.

Anthelminthics are vermifuges used in helminth infestations.

Antianemics are drugs used in the treatment of anemia.

Antibacterial agents are drugs which depress or kill bacteria.

Anticarcinogenic agents are drugs which depress the rate of growth of carcinomas.

Anticoagulants are drugs which depress the ability of blood to coagulate.

Antidotes are drugs which neutralize poisons, prevent their action, or reverse their toxic effects in the body.

Antifilarial agents are drugs which depress or kill filaria.

Antifungal agents are drugs used to control fungus infections.

Anti-infectives are drugs used to control infection.

Antiluetics are drugs used in the treatment of syphilis.

Antiparasitic agents are drugs used to control parasitic infections.

Antipruritic agents are drugs used to relieve pruritus or itching.

Antipyretics are drugs which reduce fever by a nonspecific action.

Antirickettsial agents are drugs used to control rickettsial infections.

Antiseptics are drugs which depress but do not neessarily kill pathogenic bacteria.

Antispasmodics are drugs used to relieve smooth or voluntary muscle spasm.

Antispirochetal agents are drugs used to control spirochetal infections.

Antitoxins are biologicals which neutralize bacterial toxins used in the treatment or prophylaxis of certain bacterial infections.

Antituberculous agents are drugs used in the treatment of tuberculosis.

Aperients are drugs which stimulate bowel activity.

Astringents are drugs which make the skin and mucous membranes constrict.

Bactericidal agents kill bacteria.

Bacteriostatic agents depress the activities of bacteria but do not kill them.

Carminatives are drugs used to relieve flatulence.

Cathartics are drugs which stimulate bowel activity and induce movments.

Caustics are drugs which destroy tissue on direct application.

Choleretics are drugs which stimulate the production of bile, the emptying of the gall-bladder, or which may substitute for bile.

Coagulants are drugs which accelerate the coagulation of blood.

Convulsants are drugs which induce convulsions.

Corrosives are drugs which destroy tissue.

Counterirritants are drugs which bring blood to the surface of the skin.

Decongestants are drugs used mainly to relieve swelling, especially of the nasal mucous membranes.

Demulcents are drugs which soothe and allay irritation of surfaces, the skin and mucous membranes.

Depilatories are drugs which remove hair.

Diaphoretics are drugs which stimulate sweating.

Digestants are agents which aid in digestion.

Disinfectants are drugs which destroy pathogenic bacteria.

Diuretics are drugs which increase the rate of urine formation.

Ecbolics are drugs which stimulate uterine activity.

Emetics are drugs which induce vomiting.

Emmenagogues are drugs which induce menstruation.

Emollients are drugs which soften or sooth irritated or inflamed surfaces.

Epilators are drugs which remove hair.

Escharotics are drugs which destroy tissue and form scars.

Evacuants are drugs which stimulate bowel activity and movements.
Expectorants are drugs which facilitate coughing and the production of sputum.
Fungicides are drugs which kill fungi.
Fungistatics are drugs which depress the activity of fungi but do not necessarily kill them.
Hematinics are drugs which stimulate blood formation.
Hemostatics are drugs which stop bleeding.
Hydragogues are drugs which induce watery bowel movements.
Hypnotics are drugs which help the patient fall asleep.
Hypotensives are drugs which reduce blood pressure.
Keratolytics are drugs which cause skin to peel.
Laxatives are drugs which stimulate bowel activity and movements.
Lipotropic agents are drugs related to liver function and the metabolism of lipoids.
Mesenchymal hormones are materials such as cortisone and corticotropin (ACTH) which exert a profound effect on such mesenchymal tissues as joints and muscles, and are used in the treatment of diseases of these tissues.
Miotics are drugs which constrict the pupils of the eye.
Mydriatics are drugs which dilate the pupils of the eye.
Oxytocics are drugs which stimulate uterine activity.
Parasiticides are drugs which kill parasites.
Placebos are medications without pharmacologic action which are given for purely psychologic effects.
Protectives are drugs used to prevent irritation of skin, mucous membranes or wounds.
Purgatives are drugs which stimulate bowel activity and movements.
Pyretics are drugs which induce abnormally high temperatures.
Relaxants are drugs which relax smooth or voluntary muscle spasm.
Rubifacients are drugs which increase the circulation in the skin.
Sclerosing agents are irritant drugs usually used to obliterate veins.
Sedatives are drugs which relieve anxiety and nervous tension.
Somnifacients are drugs which induce sleep.
Specifics are drugs which cure diseases, usually infectious diseases.
Stomachics stimulate the activity of the stomach.
Sudorifics are drugs which induce sweating.
Tonics are drugs which are used to increase body tone and to produce a general stimulation or sense of well-being. It is doubtful whether many drugs used for this purpose have such an action.
Vasoconstrictors are drugs which cause blood vessels to contract.
Vasodilators are drugs which cause blood vessels to relax.
Vesicants are drugs which induce blistering of the skin.

PART II

PRINCIPLES OF
THERAPEUTICS

INTRODUCTION

In the chapters which follow, diseases—their symptoms and treatment—are divided into physiologic and anatomic groups. The practical reason for this division is that for sound therapeutics we must have an understanding of the physiologic and anatomic basis of symptoms and disturbed functions. The discussions are designed to provide a basic understanding of the therapeutic actions of drugs, both in health as well as disease, how these actions may be expected to rectify disturbed functions and how they relieve symptoms. With such an understanding the nurse can anticipate the type of drug actions which may be used to advantage in certain diseases and relieve particular symptoms.

As already stated, the aims of treatment are to relieve the patient's distress, remove the cause of the disease and counteract the effects of the disease on the body and its functions. The usefulness of a drug, aided by the body and its physiologic mechanisms, depends on its ability to counteract, rectify or substitute for disturbances in function produced by the disease or to depress the patient's appreciation of the disturbance.

This section is comprised of a number of broad, general and brief discussions of physiologic and anatomic systems in the body, how they function normally, how their function is disturbed in disease, how these disturbances result in symptoms, how function is altered by drugs and how drugs may thereby relieve symptoms—in short, we present the therapeutic basis for each group of diseases.

Each section is brief. The attempt is for concise rather than extensive, detailed and exhaustive discussion. Here, as elsewhere in this book, the discussion is strictly limited to what the nurse should properly know for the practice and understanding of her profession, with no attempt to burden her with information which she may find

58

useless, needless, meaningless or difficult to handle. It is our feeling that the nurse's job is a special, unique and difficult one, and that she cannot be helped by a mass of information which does not fall into her domain, which is not practical but theoretical and which does not give meaning to the performance of her duties. The nurse administers drugs and observes their effects, but she does not order or choose them. The kind of information she needs, therefore, differs from that which may be more appropriately found in texts designed for medical students and physicians. For special and detailed considerations of a particular drug the nurse is referred to the standard medical texts on medicine, therapeutics and pharmacology. This section is not a simplification of any of these and does not attempt to replace them; it was designed to supply information about therapeutics which will help, not confuse, the nurse.

In this section drugs are used mainly by way of example and little detail is to be found here. An exception to the plan of this section is made in the case of drugs used in the cardiovascular diseases in which the detail is especially great. This is usually the case in all texts on pharmacology for many reasons. Cardiac drugs are historically the oldest of the pharmacologically effective drugs, they are drugs which have been extensively studied and about which we have a wealth of information and, finally, which are used in common and serious disease. There is also the fact that the cardiovascular system lends itself to pharmacodynamic experimentation and study. As a consequence the cardiovascular drugs serve particularly well as the basis for the understanding of the application of the principles of pharmacology to therapeutics.

Another exception is made for cortisone and corticotropin (ACTH). Although they are widely used, their actions are so unusual and they are so new that it is difficult to find summarized information about them. For this reason it was thought that special treatment was indicated.

At the end of each chapter in Part II categories of drugs used in the disorders considered in the chapter are listed. The individual drugs will be found in the Materia Medica, Part IV, under the separate headings.

9

TREATMENT OF INFECTIONS

Cause of Disease

The oldest as well as the most elusive problem in the history of the treatment of disease has been that of driving out the cause of disease. Obviously, the first information needed, and until recently lacking, was knowledge of the cause. Long before it was understood what the nature of infectious agents truly was, their infectious character had been recognized. Since it was realized that certain diseases could be transmitted from one human to another this in turn implied that some invisible disease-producing force was causing the infection. Originally the invasion of the human host and the transfer of disease to another was consigned to supernatural forces, and treatment designed accordingly. When natural and tangible forces, such as bacteria and other forms of microscopic life, were identified as the causes of many diseases it became possible to examine their characteristics and means of transmission. The problems of treatment were more clearly delineated when studies demonstrated that disease-producing micro-organisms shared many of the properties of higher forms of life.

Intestinal infestations with worms and superficial infections by insects which could be seen and identified with the naked eye were probably the first natural causes of infectious diseases to receive specific treatment. (Other diseases were assumed to be brought on by unnatural forces and were attended to by the medicine man.) The oldest medications directed against such diseases were often effective, thus supporting the contention that knowledge provides power in the treatment of disease. The mystery in most infectious disease resulted from the invisible or microscopic nature of the cause. But when the bacterial nature of some infectious diseases finally became established the same idea in treatment was applied as in the case of worms and insects. A drug was applied as directly as possible to the cause in order to destroy it. It was discovered, however, that many diseases could not be treated in this manner since the microbes had invaded deeply into the organs and tissues of the body. The problems in treating these systemic infections were far more complex than those involved in treating the relatively easily reached worms in the intestinal tract or insects on the surface of the body.

It was soon evident that drugs which killed bacteria easily in test-tube experiments might also kill human cells. If such drugs were used against a systemic invasion by bacteria the host as well as the bacteria might be killed. The patient and the bacteria, both being forms of real and active life, may be killed by similar mechanisms and by the same drugs. Thus it is that most bottles containing antiseptics are labeled, "Poison." This is for the patient to read and take notice; bacteria cannot read.

Modern Treatment of Infections

Only after many years of search for materials which were highly selective did the problem yield to the modern discoveries which we know as serums, antitoxins, chemotherapeutic agents and antibiotics—drugs which are more toxic to bacteria than patients. Early in the search for effective antibacterial drugs it was found that prophylactic measures against contamination and spread of infections might be effectively taken. Here the problem was much simpler because the bacteria had not yet invaded the host and strong agents could be used against bacteria without danger of injuring patients. Sources of contamination and dissemination can be effectively attacked by such measures as fumigation, sterilization and pasteurization. Although these developments comprised an attack against bacteria which has saved millions of lives, the large problem in medicine of finding drugs specifically effective against bacteria without being harmful to bodily organisms so that they could be used in the treatment of infectious disease, remained unsolved until recent years.

Specificity

Specificity is a special property of some chemical and biologic agents which are used against infections; it implies a high order of potency against one particular type of protoplasm, curing an infection by direct attack on the organism which causes it. The first type of specificity required is, of course, that against microbial, but not against human or animal protoplasm. This is not commonly the case with strong general antiseptics. But beyond this there are large variations in specificity. Some drugs are toxic only to a few forms of bacteria, against fungi, or worms, or protozoa, but to none others. Such highly developed specificity has great value in particular cases. When it is established that a disease is caused by one particular organism, it is then possible to use such a highly specific agent, if, indeed, one exists for that infection. On the other hand, when there is gross contamination of a wound, or the intent is to sterilize the skin which has been exposed to many varieties of microbial life, an agent with a broad spectrum of effectiveness, a general antiseptic and not a highly specific one, is needed. In general, the biologic agents tend to be highly specific in action, the chemicals of widely varying ranges of effectiveness. The choice to use one or the other type requires thought and knowledge of the nature of the infection to be attacked in this way.

This approach to the specific treatment of infectious disease as distinguished from supportive and symptomatic treatment may be divided into two categories: (1) local anti-infective measures and (2) systemic anti-infective measures. The drugs used are biologic, chemotherapeutic and antibiotic agents.

Natural Antimicrobial Agents

In an examination of the methods used to attack bacteria one must not lose sight of the fact that there are many forces operating in nature which tend to destroy bacteria. If this were not so bacteria would soon crowd all other forms of life out of existence. These natural agencies are common, so commonplace that they are frequently overlooked. Sunlight and ultra-violet light are potent forces which destroy many bacteria upon exposure. Oxygen also destroys some bacteria upon exposure. The physical forces of dilution, filtration, sedimentation and evaporation operate against bacteria found in water. Finally, time itself destroys many bacteria; many forms even if not attacked by any potent antibacterial agent will die out in time unless stimulated by especially suitable growth media. Bacteria themselves manufacture materials which are bactericidal. Thus, some bacteria stimulate the formation of bacteriophage, a material which dissolves bacteria. Other bacteria manufacture substances which we now recognize as antibiotics which inhibit or destroy other bacteria.

Aside from all these, the animal body itself possesses potent forces against bacteria. Some of these agents, as explained below (page 69) are also used therapeutically in modern medicine. Blood contains lysins, materials which dissolve bacteria, and agglutinins, materials which make bacteria clump together. White blood cells have the power of phagocytosis, engulfing and destroying bacteria. Animal tissues and fluids contain a material called lysozyme which is capable of destroying active bacteria. Digestive juices, the acid of the stomach and the alkaline juices of the intestine are potent antibacterial chemical agents and destroy bacteria ingested with food. The human skin secretes fatty acids and other substances which exert potent antibacterial action thus protecting the skin from gross infection. Human milk and colostrum contain antibacterial substances which the mother transfers to the newborn infant.

Since these potent natural antibacterial agents are in action at all times, the drugs we use to destroy bacteria must do a better job than the natural forces already there. To this end they must not only inhibit or destroy bacteria, but they must also be well tolerated by tissues. It is well to remember that potent chemicals may destroy the body's defenses as well as bacteria, and their usefulness depends on careful judgment. In the end it may prove to be more effective if the attempt with drugs is merely to inhibit bacteria rather than to destroy them. Such a procedure is less likely to destroy tissue or the body's defenses, and the latter may be able to complete what the former started.

It should be kept in mind that while it is a simple matter to sterilize an instrument, it is virtually impossible to do so with living tissue which is to remain alive. The term sterility literally means death, and any attempt at sterility of tissues with drugs is likely to produce considerable damage. The problem of killing bacteria already on or in living tissue is a completely different one from destroying the bacteria on an inanimate object. For this reason test tube experiments are never immediately applicable to medical utilization. The problems, as now to be outlined, in the treatment of infections, are far more complex than simply that of destroying micro-organisms.

Local Anti-infectives

Local anti-infective drugs are those which destroy or inhibit the growth and development of disease-producing agents by direct application to the site of infection. Their use is limited in most instances to application to the skin and easily reached mucous membranes. Most of these drugs fall into the class of local antiseptics and disinfectants, are chemical in nature and only occasionally biologic in origin.

Antiseptics and Disinfectants

There is a minor distinction, by definition, between an antiseptic and a disinfectant; the disinfectant is a substance which *kills* disease-producing bacteria whereas the antiseptic may merely *inhibit* their activity without actually killing them. In general, the same drug in one concentration is an antiseptic and in a stronger concentration is a disinfectant. In this section no distinction will be drawn between them.

Local antiseptics vary widely in potency. The *phenol coefficient* is an index of their antibacterial potency and is determined by comparing the effectiveness of an antiseptic with that of phenol (carbolic acid). The higher the phenol coefficient, the more potent than phenol the antiseptic.

The test is conducted with only one species of bacteria, *Bacillus typhosa*. The phenol coefficient, therefore, gives only limited information about the effectiveness and limitations of an antiseptic; it fails to tell about action against other bacteria, the toxicity and irritation to tissues, the effect of pus and debris. As a consequence it cannot be assumed that a particular antiseptic is safe, effective, or desirable for a particular situation on the basis of its phenol coefficient.

Antiseptics are frequently used for prophylaxis in the case of cuts, wounds, burns, accidents and in the preparation of the skin for injection and for surgery. They are also widely used in the disinfection of instruments and the decontamination of infected materials.

The effectiveness of antiseptics in the disinfection and decontamination of inanimate materials is well established, and all that is necessary is to make certain that the bacteria in question are susceptible to the agents used. There are instances in which special precautions must be taken to ascertain that the antiseptic will not destroy or injure the inanimate material being disinfected, for example, an instrument. It is a different matter, however, when the bacteria resides on the living animal.

As already pointed out chemical antiseptics tend to inhibit the natural protective mechanisms which the body provides and which may, in many instances, be even more effective than the antiseptic. In addition, chemicals which are highly toxic for microbial life are usually also highly toxic for the more complex and sensitive animal cell and, as a consequence, the local application of these chemicals may cause such tissue damage as to encourage the extension of the infection against which it is used. The final consideration in the use of chemical antiseptics is that human protoplasm, serum, pus, cellular debris, all tend to combine with the agent and thus quickly reduce its antibacterial potency. Thus, the total effect of the local application of a strong chemical to an infected area may be to depress the body's defenses, damage the infected tissues and, in the final analysis, to favor the multiplication of bacteria and the extension of the infection. For these reasons antiseptics must be carefully chosen and used; they should be chosen with regard to the specific tissue as well as the specific bacteria, and they must never be used to replace cleanliness and prophylaxis.

The possibility of hypersensitivity to the antiseptic, with subsequent skin reaction to it, is an ever-present danger. Skin reactions to iodine, for example, are not rare, and often more troublesome than the injury for which the iodine was applied. For this reason, after iodine is applied and time is given for it to work, many take the precaution of removing it with alcohol.

It is also an important fact that antiseptics take time to do their work; no antiseptic kills bacteria instantaneously. Several minutes, at least, are needed. The common practice of wetting the skin with some alcohol and plunging a hypodermic needle through it at once does not protect the patient at all, it merely makes the injection more painful by introducing alcohol under the skin. Fortunately for the patient, he almost always possesses sufficient natural antibacterial resistance to overcome the effects of this procedure. In addition, patients are protected against infection by the sterility of the solution, the needle and the syringe, for if these are contaminated, infection is more likely to result. In many instances, although bacteria on the skin may not be killed by the attempt at skin antisepsis, the rubbing combined with the cleansing action of the solvents used in the antiseptic remove a great deal of the skin soil and, in this way, prevent infection. Soil and debris depress antiseptic potency, they tend to combine with them and make them ineffectual. It is well, therefore, to cleanse any area before attempting antisepsis. This reduces the bacteria count, exposes the remaining bacteria to the antiseptic agent, and prevents exhaustion of the antiseptic by soil and debris.

Alcohol

Special mention must be made of alcohol because it is so frequently used. Alcohol is stated to exert antibacterial action at one particular concentration, namely, 70 per cent by weight. Rubbing alcohol and carelessly made up alcohol solutions, even those far stronger than 70 per cent, may be ineffective and serve only as cleansing agents. Living bacteria are often found multiplying happily in such solutions. If alcohol is to be used effectively, therefore, it must be of the proper strength; precisely 70 per cent by *weight, not by volume.*

One bit of nursing practice deserves special comment; that of placing a sterile needle between two layers of gauze wetted down with alcohol. This procedure does not make the needle sterile even when the alcohol is of the proper concentration. What is worse, is that it makes the injection far more painful than it otherwise would be because alcohol, which is highly irritant, is introduced under the skin on the surface of the needle. A far more sensible procedure is to place the sterile needle between two pads of sterile gauze.

Fungicides

Fungicides are anti-infective materials that are used against larger forms of microbial life, the fungi. Fungus infections, for the most part, are superficial but are extremely resistant to treatment with antiseptic agents. Most common among these is epidermatophytosis, or athlete's foot. It has long been recognized that the effect of strong antiseptics in many of these cases is to aggravate matters markedly. The modern tendency in treatment is to use the mildest medicaments. In recent years a group of fungicidal and fungistatic agents have been introduced all of which derive from fatty acids, undecylenic acid, propionic acid, etc. These are relatively bland, and while not always curative, rarely make matters worse. They are, in general, far more effective in holding skin fungi infections in check than any other drugs we have.

Antiprotozoal Agents

Antiprotozoal agents are used against disease caused by single celled animals. Chief among these is the ameba which causes amebic dysentery, and the malarial parasite. There is a wide range of protozoal diseases and drugs used for them. In the case of intestinal infestations, the drugs used may be considered to be of the local antiseptic variety, since many of them are given by mouth so that they reach the amebae in the intestine and kill them there directly. Other antiprotozoal drugs, such as those used in malaria, are systemic anti-infective drugs. The subject will be considered again in another section.

Antiparasitics

The antiparasitics (parasiticides) are agents used in the treatment of insect and worm infestations. In the case of the insects living on the surface of the body, local antiseptic agents, called insecticides, are especially effective. The same principles apply as in the case of local antiseptics used against bacteria, namely a drug is chosen which is far more toxic for the insect than the host. The vermifuges are considered in more detail in the section on digestive diseases (page 197).

Urinary Antiseptics

The modern urinary antiseptics are taken by mouth and circulate through the bloodstream, and they may be properly considered to be systemically acting drugs. The older urinary antiseptics were often injected directly and acted as local antiseptics. They are discussed in the section on diseases of the urinary system (page 233).

Skin Antiseptics

Skin antisepsis for surgery is a special problem and one which has long vexed the surgeon. The limitations are clearly recognized by him and, to a large extent, it is accepted that the measures taken merely reduce the number of living bacteria on the skin. At the present time two new groups of materials are widely used, the detergents such as phemerol and the antiseptic soaps such as pHisoderm. The latter have an unusual property of inducing a relatively persistent antibacterial state which makes them especially useful for the scrubbing of the skin and the surgeon's hands. The problem of skin antisepsis, as it affects the dermatologist, is discussed on page 257.

Systemic Anti-infectives

The systemic anti-infectives are drugs which taken internally are absorbed and circulate through the bloodstream, thus reaching the site of infection in the tissues and organs. Virtually all of these drugs are specifics, curing the infection by attacking only the organism which causes it. Biologicals, chemotherapeutic drugs and antibiotics are the three main varieties of specifics; they can be used against micro-organisms (bacteria, spirochetes, viruses, rickettsial bodies, protozoa, fungi), regardless of whether the infection can be reached by the local application of drugs. In most cases of infection, the disease is diffuse and only by such an approach is specific therapy possible. For example, it is impossible to treat such a widespread infection as syphilis by any other means than with a drug which diffuses throughout the body.

Biologicals

The biologicals comprise a large group of materials classified as vaccines and serums. They are all anti-infective in purpose, used either to stimulate the body to produce its own defenses (antibodies) against infections, or to supply antibodies derived from another body, animal or human, when the diseased body cannot produce its own quickly enough or in sufficient amount. Thus the biologicals are agents which, in one way or another, make use of animal biologic defense mechanisms for the attack on infections.

Vaccines

Vaccines are living, attenuated, or dead disease-producing micro-organisms or their toxins. They are used solely to stimulate the body to produce its own specific antibodies by producing a controlled, attenuated, or simulated disease reaction. In some instances, stock bacteria, grown in the laboratory are used to make the vaccine. This is the case with typhoid vaccine. These are usually called stock vaccines. In other instances, the particular strain of bacteria is obtained from the patient himself, and a so-called autogenous vaccine is made from it. Vaccines often are highly specific in their action, and often effective against only one strain of a species of bacteria.

This type of therapy, so frequently used years ago, has largely been discarded. This has been due to the poor results of accumulated experience with autogenous and stock vaccines. There has always been reason to question the validity of the concept of vaccine therapy in the treatment of infections already established, since there is no adequate explanation why dead bacteria injected in the form of a vaccine should stimulate a patient to produce antibodies when the same bacteria, already in his body in a living and active form, have failed to do so. There is also the consideration that once the vaccine is given there is usually a delay of some weeks before appreciable amounts of antibody are produced; a delay not permissible in the case of most acute infections.

On the other hand, vaccines are important and effective agents for prophylaxis. The immunity they induce is persistent, often lasting for years, but, as already indicated, it often takes weeks to develop. The smallpox and typhoid vaccines are the best known examples. Unfortunately, not all vaccines are effective in stimulating immunity.

Another field of vaccine therapy of decreasing popularity is the use of vaccines in a nonspecific manner to stimulate the resistance against a disease not related to the bacteria used in making up the vaccine. Thus, typhoid vaccine may be given to a patient with a rheumatic infection in the hope that the reaction to the vaccine will, in some way, stimulate resistance to disease in general, and that this will include the rheumatic infection. Another example of much the same practice is the use of the so-called "cold" vaccine. This is composed of a mixture of bacteria not at all related to the virus which causes the cold, and is used with the hope that if it does not increase the resistance to a cold it may at least increase resistance to infections by secondary invaders.

In many instances vaccines are primarily used to induce a febrile reaction. Typhoid vaccine induces a high fever in many patients. Some feel that such febrile reactions may increase general resistance to disease, but there is considerable debate whether this is ever true, and if it is, whether the fever induced by an unrelated organism can be of any value. If there is any value in such reactions, the injections of milk and milk proteins, also used to induce febrile reactions, should be just as effective as that of bacterial vaccines.

Toxoids

Toxoids are a special category of vaccine which are made, not from bacteria, but from attenuated or weakened bacterial toxins. They increase resistance only against the toxin used, and are given only for prophylaxis, never in treatment. Patients who have been previously immunized against the toxin, may benefit immediately after exposure by rapid "boosting," but never once the symptoms of infection develop. The best known of the toxoids are the diphtheria and tetanus toxoids. These induce a specific but modified disease reaction which, in each case, induces the development of the specific antitoxins and thus increases resistance to these infections. This type of immunity is relatively persistent.

It used to be felt that the stimulant properties of vaccines and toxoids were antagonistic and that they were best given individually and at widely separated times so that each material had ample opportunity to induce its own kind of immunity. It is now well established that this is not at all necessary, and that much time and pain may be spared by injecting mixed vaccines and stimulating several immunities simultaneously.

Serums

Serums are blood extracts or concentrates which contain the specific antibodies against disease and are used to provide the patient quickly with an immunity or resistance to a disease. Such passively acquired resistance is always short-lived but has the advantage of being immediate, and for that reason is especially useful in the treatment of disease or in prophylaxis after exposure. The functions of serums and vaccines are, therefore, clearly different. The vaccine stimulates the host to produce his own immunity, which is slow to develop but long lasting. The serum acting more like a chemotherapeutic agent, supplies immediate offense against an infection, an effect which, however, is of short duration.

Serums may be obtained from man or animals. In the case of the animal the disease is produced in a modified or attenuated form. After the animal recovers fully, some of his blood, which contains the specific antibodies the animal formed when he cured himself of the induced disease, is drawn off and the serum separated. This can then be concentrated or further purified. Human or convalescent serum is obtained from the blood of patients who have recovered from diseases which they acquired by themselves.

Unfortunately not all diseases produce antibodies which may be recovered from the blood of man or animals in this way. This is one of the serious limits of this form of therapy; otherwise serum therapy would long have been the answer to all infectious disease. Another, and sometimes a very serious drawback is that animal serums tend to be highly allergenic, and may cause severe allergic reactions. Attempts, therefore, have been made to reduce the serums to purified antibodies.

Pooled Serum

Mixed or pooled human serum and plasma is a mixture of specimens taken from many humans, usually in the collection of blood for war and civilian casualties. Patients who have had specific diseases are not selected, but the pooled blood represents such a variety of specimens that it always contains many kinds of antibodies and may be useful as an anti-infective agent.

Serum Globulin

Serum globulin (gamma globulin) is a purified product of the pooled serum which appears to contain most of the anti-infective antibodies in the pooled blood. Such a concentrated antibody material may be very effective in the treatment of a number of infectious diseases such as measles, whooping cough, etc.

Antitoxins are serums which contain antibodies specific against the toxins produced by bacteria, rather than against the bacteria. The most common antitoxins are those for diphtheria, tetanus and gas gangrene infections.

Storage of Biologicals

The storage of biologicals usually presents more of a problem than that of chemical drugs. Most biologic agents deteriorate rapidly unless kept at the proper temperature, usually around 3° to 4° C.; they will still deteriorate at this temperature but much more slowly. The nurse should examine the package in every case to find the proper storage conditions and expiration date. All materials not properly stored should be discarded regardless of expiration date, and if the date has been passed, regardless of storage precautions.

Chemotherapeutic Drugs

Chemotherapeutic drugs are chemical agents which may be used to cure infectious disease by destroying the cause. The most useful of these are those which may be taken internally and, after circulating through the body, exert a diffuse anti-infective action within the tissues and organs of the body. Prior to 1909 there was only one really effective specific remedy in medicine, quinine for malaria; mercury and bismuth used for syphilis and chaulmoogra oil for leprosy were effective only to a limited degree. In 1909 Paul Ehrlich introduced the arsenical drug, arsphenamine (Salvarsan, 606) for the cure of syphilis. This was the first synthetic drug used for what Ehrlich termed, systemic antisepsis. It represented the result of many years of search for a drug which was so much less toxic for the patient than for the cause of syphilis *(Treponema pallida)* that it could safely be given to humans in effective doses. In the case of most drugs tested in animals, the reverse was true. Unfortunately salvarsan was effective only against syphilis and no other important infection.

It was hoped that this feat, namely, systemic antisepsis, would open a new field in drugs and that as much could be accomplished for other diseases. The first success in the case of syphilis was followed by an intensive search for other specific chemical agents for other infectious diseases, but the results were not rewarding. By 1932 only a handful were found, and these were effective only in some statistically unimportant diseases. In 1932, quinine and salvarsan were still the only important chemotherapeutic drugs.

Sulfonamides

The effect of the sulfonamide drugs on streptococcal infection was discovered in 1932. It was found that they could be safely and effectively used in a wide variety of common and serious infections: pneumonia, puerperal sepsis, streptococcus infections, gonorrhea, meningitis, urinary tract infections. Thus the field of chemotherapeusis which had virtually been abandoned because of lack of success was reopened. Since then, fully 5000 derivatives of sulfanilamide have been synthesized and screened in an attempt to find better and more effective sulfa drugs. So thorough was this search that it is probable that we now have the most effective and safest sulfa drugs we are likely to have.

When the sulfa drugs were introduced they were of the first importance in medicine. They have been relegated to the therapeutic background only because the newer antibiotics have still greater advantages in many diseases. Nevertheless, there are still some important diseases such as meningitis, and situations in which sulfonamides are the drugs of choice; their place in modern medicine is still unique.

The chief difficulties with sulfa drugs are their toxic effects which necessitate careful and constant attention. Occasionally, in a case of idiosyncrasy, a blood dyscrasia develops which may be extremely serious or even fatal. To avoid such reactions, frequent blood counts must be made. Most of the drugs are also relatively insoluble and when given in large and effective doses they tend to crystallize as they are excreted into the urine. When the crystals form in the substance of the kidney they may cause obstruction or serious kidney damage. The urine is usually kept alkaline to avoid such renal reactions, for the sulfa drugs are far more soluble in alkaline than acid urine.

Another device which may help to prevent these renal reactions is the practice of mixing two or three varieties of sulfa drugs, the sum totaling the prescribed dose. Such combinations are effective therapeutically and, at the same time, are more easily dissolved in the urine than the same total amount of any one of the combination. Because sulfa drugs vary in solubility this physical fact may be the basis of the selection of a particular drug. In urinary tract infections and in infants, the more soluble sulfa drugs such as sulfacetamide and sulfasoxazole are especially likely to be used.

Differences in the effectiveness of sulfa drugs against various pathogenic bacteria have been suggested by some physicians. In general, these differences are not a matter of great practical importance in the selection of the drug for a particular infection. Much more important is the toxicity for the patient, its solubility, its absorption and its excretion; these usually determine which sulfa drug will be used in a particular situation.

With the discovery of such effective chemotherapeutic agents as the sulfa drugs the problem was to find the best possible method of using them. The answer to this problem was the establishment of a relatively new approach to medication: the maintenance of a constant effective therapeutic concentration of the drug in the bloodstream. This is especially important therapeutically because the level of the sulfa drug in the blood stream, being the same as that in the other tissues and organs of the body, serves as an index of therapeutic effectiveness in organs and tissues. The chemical test of drug in the blood is, therefore, used in determining and scheduling dosage. In order to maintain constant levels, the drug must be given relatively frequently and round-the-clock medication is usually the rule. Prior to the sulfa drugs the use of round-the-clock medication schedules was rare because drugs were not effective enough to justify awakening the patient.

Early experiences with sulfa drugs saw them applied topically to wounds, the skin, the site of surgical procedures, etc. While this is an effective antibacterial procedure, there is good evidence that it retards healing and that systemic use which does not retard healing is just as effective for local infections. As a consequence topical use of the sulfa drugs has decreased.

Antibacterial Action of Sulfonamides

A few words may be profitably spent on the nature of the antibacterial action of sulfa drugs. They do not kill bacteria directly but appear to inhibit them, and the completion of the cure is accomplished by the patient himself. As a consequence, cure of a disease with sulfa drugs is likely to leave the patient with some immunity against the infection. This is to be contrasted to experiences with some of the antibiotics such as penicillin, which appears to kill disease-producing bacteria directly, and hence, following its use the patient may have little or no resistance against the infection just eradicated.

The means by which the sulfa drugs inhibit bacteria is very interesting and has opened up a new field in theoretic pharmacology, that of chemical analogues. The action of the sulfa drugs depends on their close resemblance to para-aminobenzoic acid, more conveniently called PABA, a vitamin material which is essential to many bacteria. Some bacteria are apparently not able to distinguish between the sulfa drug and PABA, and when the former is present, they attempt to use it instead of the latter. Because of this error in judgment, their activity is sharply reduced and they become victims of the body's defenses. The effectiveness of the sulfa drugs in therapy can be sharply diminished by administration of PABA, and even procaine, which resembles PABA closely in chemical structure.

The disease-producing bacteria which are not affected by the sulfa drugs are apparently those which can manufacture the PABA themselves, are perceptive enough to tell the difference between PABA and sulfa drugs, or do not require PABA for their life processes.

Antimalarial Drugs

The newer drugs for the treatment of malaria form another important group of chemotherapeutic agents. Malaria is probably one of the greatest of the world's problems in infectious disease; it disables and kills more people than any other single infection. Quinine has long been known for malaria, and while it is effective, it requires long and persistent use, does not cure all forms of malaria, does not eradicate the carrier state and is relatively expensive. Relapses after treatment with quinine are common and many who are apparently cured of the disease with this drug carry and disseminate it and suffer from relapses for the rest of their lives.

Better drugs for malaria have long been sought. Research during the late war provided several new and effective antimalarlial drugs (described in the Materia Medica) which have helped to simplify the problems attending both prophylaxis and treatment of malaria, and these have largely displaced quinine in all aspects of the treatment of malaria. New and more effective drugs for some of the less common tropical diseases have also developed from research made necessary by the introduction of our troops into tropical areas.

Heavy Metals

The heavy metals, arsenic, antimony, mercury and bismuth in organic forms, have long been established as chemotherapeutic agents, especially for some tropical diseases. With the exception of a few, their importance has fallen sharply with the introduction of the newer chemotherapeutic agents and antibiotics. Penicillin, for example, has virtually replaced the arsenicals, mercury and bismuth in the treatment of syphilis which, prior to recent years was the most important disease for which these metals were used. In cases of syphilis with hypersensitivity to penicillin, the arsenicals are still used, but the usefulness of these metals as a group is now largely in the field of tropical diseases. In this area there have been new and less toxic forms, which have largely replaced the older forms of the same metals, especially arsenic and antimony compounds.

Antitubercular Drugs

At the time of this writing much newspaper publicity has attended a new chemotherapeutic agent for tuberculosis, isonicotinic acid hydrazide. If the early newspaper reports are fully warranted, a most important addition to therapy has been made. The chronic nature of tuberculosis is such, however, that valid judgments cannot be established quickly and, therefore, much more time must elapse before anything definite can be said about the reported cures and the late toxic effects of the drug.

One of the chief sources of concern about this drug is whether it will have the same characteristics which so seriously limit the value of the antibiotic, streptomycin, in this disease, namely the rapid development of bacterial resistance to the drug. There is already evidence that bacterial resistance to isonicotinic acid hydrazide develops quickly and unless it is properly used its value will be sharply reduced. This is the reason that a better drug than streptomycin is needed and has been sought for tuberculosis. It may turn out after study, that isonicotinic acid hydrazide or one of its derivatives is the drug of choice for the treatment of tuberculosis or that some combination is the most effective procedure, but at present this agent is at best merely an adjunct in the standard treatment. As yet there is no evidence for it as a complete cure of the disease. There is indication that this drug may be best used in combination with streptomycin or para-amino salicylic acid (PAS).

Antibiotics

The antibiotics are materials which are formed by living microorganisms which are toxic to other species of microbial life. It may be conjectured that the original purpose of these materials was that of defense, the microbe making a substance which kept other microbes from pushing it out of existence.

Many if not most microbes develop such antibiotic substances, but of the large number of antibiotics which have been isolated since the introduction of penicillin, very few are useful in medicine. Most of these cannot be used because of toxicity to humans. Of the remaining antibiotic materials, almost all are ineffective against the microbes which cause disease in man. Thus, of the thousands which have been isolated and screened only a handful remain which combine the rare qualities of effectiveness against human disease and safety for human use. These two aspects, effectiveness and safety must always be considered for every new antibiotic contemplated for human use. And the fact that antibiotics are likely to be highly toxic for man must always be remembered. Our wonderful experiences with the effective and extremely safe penicillin are not to be taken to apply to all antibiotics.

Most antibiotics which are used in medicine at this time are derived from molds, especially those which occur naturally in the soil. There are a few antibiotics, and not the especially important ones, which are derived from bacteria. The bacterially derived antibiotics tend to be highly toxic for humans when taken systemically and, for the most part, are used externally only. This does not, of course, imply that at a later date antibiotics may not be derived from bacteria which are entirely safe for internal use.

Penicillin

The first and by far the most important of all antibiotics is penicillin. It is the most potent antibacterial substance yet known, destroying some susceptible species of bacteria in such minute dilutions as one part in 50 million. It *kills* bacteria directly, in the test tube as well as in man, yet, surprisingly enough, penicillin is outstanding for its lack of toxicity for man. Astronomical numbers of units may be given without ill effect. On the other hand, it is a highly allergenic material and most of the troublesome reactions come from allergic rather than strictly toxic reactions. Penicillin cures many common serious infections in man, pneumonia, streptococcal and staphylococcal infections, osteomyelitis, puerperal sepsis, meningitis, syphilis, gonorrhea and others. In general penicillin is effec-

tive only against bacteria, usually cocci, the outstanding exception
being the treponema of syphilis.

Streptomycin

Streptomycin is a more recent antibiotic than penicillin, and
while it is not as potent as penicillin in pneumonia and a few
other diseases in which either may be used, it is effective against
many which penicillin does not affect at all. Chief among the latter
are the common infections of the urinary tract, *Bacillus coli* infections, Friedländer's pneumonia, *Hemophilus influenzae* meningitis, tuberculosis and leprosy.

A serious limitation with streptomycin is that bacteria quickly
acquire an ability to resist it, that is to say, resistant bacterial forms
quickly develop. This resistance is transmitted to the progeny of
the bacteria, so that resistance once acquired is a permanent property of that strain of infectious organism. Unless a disease is
promptly   cured with streptomycin, therefore, a resistant form
quickly replaces the original form, and the streptomycin then becomes completely ineffective. This applies not only to tuberculosis,
a fact which seriously limits its usefulness, but also to all other disease in which streptomycin is effective. It is a prominent feature
of streptomycin and, although it may also appear in the case
of other antibiotics, it is not nearly as important or as constant.

It has been found that para-amino salicylic acid, often called
PAS, also has an antitubercular action. When used together with
streptomycin not only is the antitubercular action increased but the
tendency to development of resistance is markedly delayed. At the
present time streptomycin is used together with PAS in the treatment of tuberculosis.

In addition, streptomycin, and to a lesser degree its derivative,
dihydrostreptomycin, is a drug with serious toxic potentialities. Disturbances in vestibular function are common and permanent loss to
the sense of equilibrium has not been rare. Kidney damage also
occurs but is less common. Deafness may sometimes develop. Streptomycin is not a drug to be taken lightly; it is to be used only in
conditions which justify the risk of taking it. Once used, dosage

must be effective so that the disease is cured before streptomycin resistance develops.

Other Antibiotics

A group of antibiotics (the tetracyclines, chloramphenicol, erythromycin, and carbomycin) all derived from different species of streptomyces but with closely related therapeutic properties have recently been introduced into medical practice. These are sometimes designated as the broad-spectrum antibiotics because of the wide range of their effectiveness. They are effective against many diseases sensitive to penicillin (not including syphilis) and, in addition, many others of importance. They are the only antibiotics which are effective against some viruses and rickettsial infections. There is evidence of effectiveness of tetracycline in amebic dysentery. In general, they are nontoxic and the most serious difficulty with them is gastrointestinal upsets. These may often be avoided by giving the dose together with sodium bicarbonate or directly after eating. An interesting reaction in some cases is the development of a peri-anal or vulvar rash, due to the growth of micro-organisms (mainly monilia), which tolerate the broad-spectrum antibiotics and flourish in the relatively sterile field which is produced by the use of these antibiotics.

At the very time of this writing some publicity has been given to blood dyscrasias which have developed after the use of chloramphenicol. Whether there is a cause-and-effect relationship is not yet established, but it seems probable that in hypersensitive cases it may actually be the case. As matters now stand, this drug is to be used only when no other antibiotic will suffice.

A few other antibiotics such as bacitracin, polymyxin, neomycin, tyrothricin, are useful but not of the first importance. For the most part these materials are too toxic for anything but external use, and are used internally only in very special situations. All of these antibiotics are further described in the Materia Medica.

Choosing the Antibiotic

In general, because of its great potency and low order of toxicity, penicillin is the antibiotic of choice in all infections in which it is effective. When the cause of an infection is responsive to only one antibiotic, obviously that particular substance is the one to be used, but when there is a choice between penicillin and another material, and no hypersensistivity to penicillin is known, penicillin is the drug of choice. In cases in which precise information as to cause is not available, the broad-spectrum antibiotics may be used. This group may also prove to be the one of choice as prophylactic agents against many diseases.

There has been a tendency to give combinations of antibiotics in those cases in which the cause of infection is either not known or in which the infection fails to respond to one drug alone. In some instances combinations are very effective, but in others an antagonism between them may occur. Combinations, therefore, can be used only after careful consideration.

Mode of Administration

The mode of administration of antibiotics is an important practical matter. As in the case of the chemotherapeutic agents, it is usually desirable to maintain effective amounts of the antibiotics in the blood and tissues at all times. In early experiences with penicillin, the material had to be injected intramuscularly at frequent intervals because it was relatively rapidly eliminated. With the recent development of penicillin in suspension and procaine penicillin, the slowly absorbed or depot forms of the drug, such frequent dosage is not required. Because of the slow absorption enough may be injected at one time to provide a depot of penicillin to last for 48 or even 72 hours. This has made possible penicillin treatment with injection daily or every other day instead of every few hours, as was formerly the practice.

Penicillin may also be given effectively by mouth, but since about four-fifths of the amount taken by mouth is destroyed, the usual oral dose is about five times the intramuscular dose. Since the introduction of the effective and convenient depot forms of penicillin, the oral form is not as popular as before but it still has convenience for some cases. Most physicians, however, will not depend on oral administration for urgently ill patients.

Various forms of penicillin itself have been introduced. The original preparation of penicillin was an amorphous material, a mixture of several types designated as F, G, K and X. In order to insure constancy of potency the tendency has been to crystallize the penicillin and to separate the various forms. Today virtually all crystalline penicillin sold is of the G form. This may be in the form of sodium, potassium, or calcium salts, although the sodium salts are by far the most commonly used.

Procaine penicillin, a chemical combination between penicillin G and procaine, is widely used as a slowly absorbed form. After the injection of procaine penicillin, the penicillin is slowly liberated and absorbed, then operating in the same way as when plain penicillin is injected. Benzethacil (bicillin) is another slowly absorbed form of penicillin which has just been introduced. Still another recently introduced form, neo-pentil, is reported to have a tendency to concentrate in the lungs, and is, therefore, prescribed for pulmonary infection. Such a wide variety of forms are not yet available in the other antibiotics.

Finally there are chemical derivatives of penicillin which have been created in an attempt to obtain a less allergenic form which may be used in those patients who have exhibited allergic reactions to the standard forms of penicillin. To some extent this has been accomplished with penicillin O, a form just as effective as the regular penicillin but less allergenic and safe in patients who have already shown allergic manifestations after penicillin.

The broad-spectrum antibiotics may be effectively used by mouth because of good absorption and relatively slow elimination; doses taken every 4 hours maintain effective concentrations in the body. Because of serious difficulties in perfecting parenteral preparations of these drugs, this form of administration has not been frequently used. At the present time, however, there are parenteral preparations which may be used safely and effectively in situations in which the oral route may not be used.

In special instances antibiotics may be administered directly at the site of infection, into the spinal canal, a joint cavity, a lung abscess, etc. This is made possible by the numerous pharmaceutical preparations available, such as ointments, aerosol sprays, douches, lozenges and nasal sprays.

Manufacture of Antibiotics

All but one of the antibiotics in actual use are made by living micro-organisms grown in the manufacturer's laboratory and extracted from the growth media, purified and prepared for commercial use. Chloramphenicol is the exception; it is the only antibiotic which is now synthesized on a commercial scale. Although the chemical structure of many of the others has been established, the processes involved are far too complex to make synthesis commercially practicable.

Bacteriophage

Bacteriophage is a material which is formed by some bacteria in the media in which they grow and is capable of dissolving the very bacteria which stimulated its development. In this way it is completely different from the antibiotics which are well tolerated by the microbes which form it. Just how bacteriophage is developed is not known, but its effect in the laboratory is impressive as it literally dissolves bacteria. When this phenomenon was first noted about forty years ago hopes were raised that this effect could be reproduced in man; that disease could be cured by the administration of the specific bacteriophage which would dissolve the bacteria in the host. This, unfortunately, rarely proves to be the case, and now that we have effective and dependable chemotherapeutic agents and antibiotics, bacteriophage is seldom heard from.

Warning

A special note of warning, sounded earlier in regard to the misuse of drugs, may well be repeated here. We stand in danger of losing our so-called miracle drugs through improper and indiscriminate use. As we have seen with streptomycin, bacteria may acquire resistance to other antibiotics and chemotherapeutic agents. The only special feature in the case of streptomycin is the exceeding rapidity with which resistant strains appear. This resistance is a permanent feature of the bacteria; once acquired that strain of bacteria continues to be resistant to the particular drug. The other danger in indiscriminate use relates to the development of allergies. Humans tend to develop allergic states after exposure to particular drugs no

Table 1—Common Infections and Agents Effective in Treatment

Disease or Infection	Agents of Choice
Actinomycosis	Penicillin
Amebic dysentery	The tetracyclines
Anthrax	Penicillin
Bacillary dysentery	The tetracyclines or sulfonamides
Bacterial endocarditis	Differs with organisms
Brucellosis	Dihydrostreptomycin and broad-spectrum antibiotics
Chancroid	Dihydrostreptomycin
Cholera	Combination of dihydrostreptomycin and sulfonamide
Common cold	None
Diphtheria	Combination of penicillin and antitoxin
Erysipelas	Penicillin
Gonorrhea	Penicillin
Granuloma inguinale	Dihydrostreptomycin
Lymphogranuloma venereum	The tetracyclines or penicillin
Malaria	Chloroguanide, chloroquin, pentaquin, quinacrine, primaquin, camoquin, quinine
Meningitis	
Meningococcus	Combination of sulfonamide and penicillin
Pneumococcus	Combination of sulfonamide and penicillin
H. influenzae	Combination of sulfonamide, dihydrostreptomycin and serum
Others	Differs with organism
Pneumonia	
Pneumococcus	Penicillin
H. influenzae	Dihydrostreptomycin, the tetracyclines
Klebsiella	Dihydrostreptomycin, the tetracyclines
Virus (atypical)	The tetracyclines; questionable value
Psittacosis	The tetracyclines
Q Fever	The tetracyclines
Relapsing fever	Penicillin
Rickettsial infections	The tetracyclines
Scarlet fever	Penicillin
Spotted fever	The tetracyclines
Staphylococcus	Penicillin, erythromycin, or carbomycin
Streptococcus	Penicillin
Subacute bacterial endocarditis	Penicillin, but differs with organisms
Syphilis	Penicillin
Tetanus	Penicillin and antitoxin
Trachoma	The tetracyclines
Tuberculosis	Combination of dihydrostreptomycin and PAS, or isonicotinic acid hydrazide
Tularemia	Dihydrostreptomycin, the tetracyclines
Typhoid fever	The tetracyclines
Typhus fever	The tetracyclines
Urinary tract infections	Differs with organisms

Table 1—Continued

Disease or Infection	Agents of Choice
Vincent's angina	Penicillin
Whooping cough	The tetracyclines
Yaws	Penicillin

matter whether the drug is useful or not. Thus a patient may develop an allergy after receiving an antibiotic which does not happen to be useful for the particular condition for which it was applied. Then, at a later date, when the antibiotic is urgently needed the patient may not be able to tolerate it.

There is a real possibility, therefore, that by indiscriminate use and improper dosage, many patients will not be able to tolerate the miracle drugs and many bacteria will become resistant to them. The only way to avoid such a disaster is to use the drugs only when they are clearly indicated, and at that time, to use them in full and adequate dosage until the disease is completely cured. A list of diseases or infections, indicating the drugs which are effective in their treatment, is found in table 1.

New anti-infective drugs will continue to be introduced, many proving to be useful. But it is well to withhold judgment about them until it is proved that the drug will induce a permanent cure, not a temporary remission, and that it will not turn out to be too toxic for most patients.

Drugs Used in Treatment of Infections

Antibiotics
Antifilarials
Antileutics
Antimalarials
Antiprotozoals
Antiseptics (local, intestinal
   and urinary)
Antirickettsials

Antituberculars
Chemotherapeutics
Fungicides
Parasiticides
Serums
Toxoids
Vaccines
Vermifuges

Study Questions

1. What is the chief problem involved in finding agents which can be used in the treatment of infections in man?

2. What are some natural and physical forces which may be utilized to combat infections?

3. What are the two major groups of local anti-infective drugs, and in what ways do they differ?

4. What are three significant factors which influence the effectiveness of local anti-infective agents in man?

5. Indicate the practical significance of each, from a nursing standpoint.

6. What is a *specific* anti-infective agent?

7. Into what three groups may these be divided?

8. How do they differ?

9. How do each of the following differ: vaccine, toxoid, serum, antitoxin?

10. What specific precautions must be taken in the storage of most biologicals?

11. What are some of the specific disadvantages of the sulfonamides and how may these be overcome?

12. What is the nature of action and effectiveness of the sulfonamides?

13. What are certain disadvantages in the use of quinine as an antimalarial agent?

14. In the prolonged use of broad spectrum antibiotics, monilia infections may develop. How is this believed to come about?

15. What do we mean by "depot" preparations? Give examples.

16. Indiscriminate use of antibiotics requires what special warnings? What is the significance in each case?

10

TREATMENT OF
NERVOUS SYSTEM DISORDERS

The nervous system which controls the activities of the body consists of the brain, the spinal cord and a complex system of nerves. The organs and activities of the body controlled by the nervous system are: (1) *voluntarily moving parts,* the muscles and joints of limbs and trunk; (2) *organs which move automatically or involuntarily,* the diaphragm, intestinal tract, gall-bladder, ureters, urinary bladder, uterus, heart and arteries; (3) *secretory organs,* the endocrine, salivary and digestive organs, the sweat and tear glands; (4) *a variety of conscious sensorial functions,* sight, pain, hearing, odor, taste, heat, vibration, touch, balance; (5) *mental processes,* thinking, speech, writing; (6) *emotional reactions,* joy, fear, anger and so forth.

The nervous system may also be divided into the two main categories of central nervous system and autonomic nervous system. The central nervous system consists of parts of the brain and spinal cord, and nerves which are mainly concerned with conscious function. The autonomic nervous system consists of parts of the brain and spinal cord, and nerves which are concerned with automatic or vegetative functions of the body. These nerves regulate the activities of internal organs, gland secretions, heart, arterial tone, respiration, etc. The brain is able to control the entire body and its functions through the spinal cord and nerves, its pathways of communication. These connect the centrally placed brain with every functioning part of the body. Nerves are of two types, those which bring messages or nerve impulses back to the brain from their origins elsewhere in the body, and those which conduct messages or impulses arising in the brain to distant parts of the body.

The symptoms which may arise from a disturbance in so complex

and widespread a system as this are varied and often present the
physician with serious problems in diagnosis as well as treatment.
The symptoms here discussed have been selected because of their
importance as therapeutic problems.

Pain

Although pain is a symptom which may develop in disease of
any system in the body, its mediation, appreciation and often its relief involves the nervous system. It is a symptom which is often urgently in need of relief; in some cases relief of pain may become
the most pressing problem in treatment. It is probably the symptom
for which more medication is applied than any other in medicine.
There are many drugs which effectively relieve most types of pain;
some of these are about as old as medicine itself, yet the problem
of their proper application is not one which is simply solved. The
complications arise in the numerous varieties of pain, variations
in patient tolerance to pain and response to drugs and the many
other facets to the problem of the relief of pain. The too ready, too
frequent and too heroic attempts to relieve pain have had consequences more serious than the painful condition itself. A program
for the relief of pain which is not well thought out may lead to addiction, habituation, tolerance or serious intoxication.

Relief of Pain

There are two fundamental approaches to the relief of pain. How
it is actually done depends on the nature of the illness, the quality
of pain, its severity, probable duration, and the nature of the drug
which is required to relieve it. The approaches used are as follows:
(1) Anesthesia. In this state all pain perception is completely oblit-
erated as with ether anesthesia for an operation. (2) Analgesia. In
this state pain perception is depressed but coma or anesthesia are
not induced. Examples of the latter are the use of morphine for a
patient with a broken leg and the taking of an aspirin tablet for the
relief of headache.

Anesthetics

Drugs which relieve or prevent pain by interfering with the

patient's ability to perceive sensory stimuli are called anesthetics. There are two categories of anesthetics, general and local. General anesthesia obliterates the patient's ability to perceive sensory stimuli from all parts of the body by depressing his cerebral functions to the degree that he falls into a deep sleep or coma from which he cannot be aroused even by the most painful stimulation. Local anesthesia alters or blocks the nerves by applying anesthetic drugs directly to them, so that they cannot conduct pain sensations to the brain. While the patient cannot appreciate pain in the area blocked by this procedure, he has normal sensations and responses elsewhere in his body.

General Anesthetics

Inhalation anesthetics: One of the two types of general anesthetics is that which is administered by inhalation as, for example, ether. The gas or inhalation anesthetics are absorbed from the lungs into the bloodstream, depress cerebral function and induce deep sleep. Usually these anesthetics are largely excreted by the lungs. Effects develop quickly and excretion is almost as rapid. Thus the depth of anesthesia can be varied from moment to moment by changing the rate of administration of the gas. Inhalation anesthesia, an example of the administration of a drug by inhalation, is one of the most flexible types of drug administration: effects can be intensified or decreased at a moment's notice. This is an especially important feature since general anesthesia represents a profound degree of drug action on the brain. There are situations after induction in which it is vitally important to decrease the depth of anesthesia quickly, perhaps because of a cardiac or respiratory emergency. Only in the case of inhalation anesthesia is it possible to do this. But in hand with its flexibility is the fact that it also requires the constant attention of the anesthetist to maintain a constant level of anesthesia.

Stages of Anesthesia

The depth or degree of general anesthesia is usually designated by stages which are determined by the state of the central nervous system and reflex activity. These are merely devices used by the

ACTION OF GENERAL ANESTHESIA (ETHER)

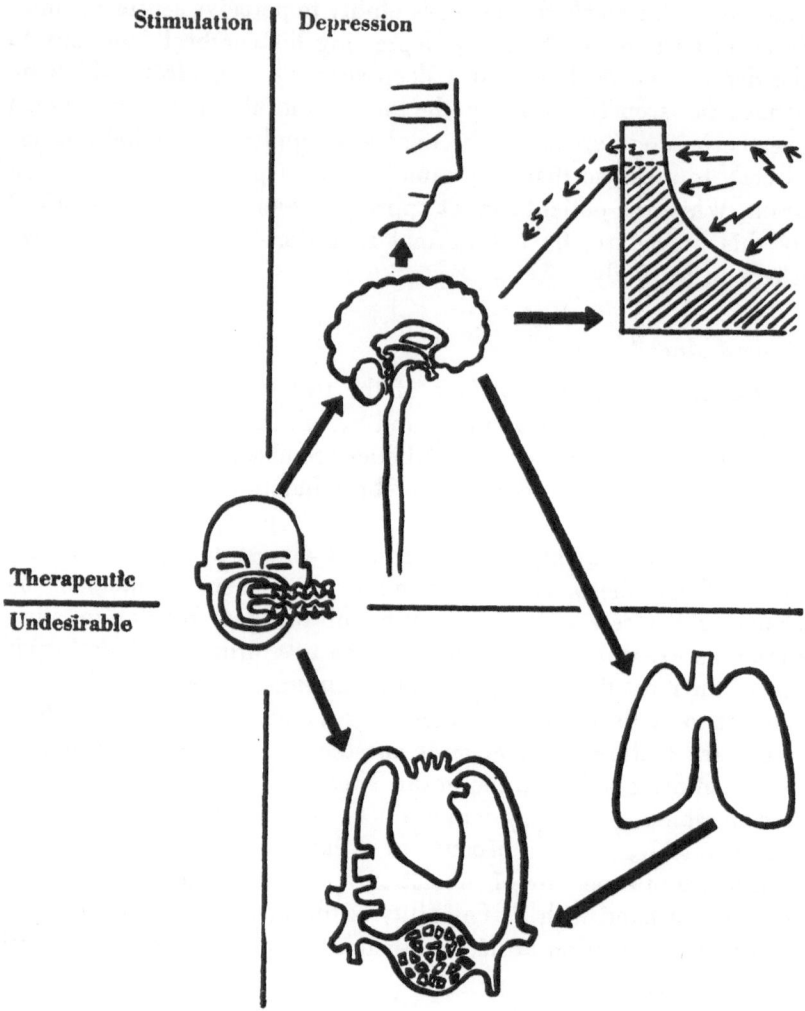

Fig. 1—General anesthetics mainly exert depressant actions. The therapeutic effect consists of depression of the brain which induces sleep, and depression of pain appreciation (elevates pain threshold). The toxic effects consist of a depressant action on the cardiovascular system and the respiratory center.

anesthetist to indicate the condition of the patient and whether the state of anesthesia is such that surgery may proceed or the patient is dangerously intoxicated. The depressant action of most general anesthetics proceeds in much this order: mental processes, coordination, sensation, motor function and, finally, vital vegetative functions. The distinction between stages of anesthesia is never clearly delineated since one stage passes into the next without special incident to mark it, making it often difficult to detect the end of one stage and the beginning of the next.

There is no uniformity in description of the stages of anesthesia. The simplest classification divides anesthesia into four stages: (I) analgesia or irritation, (II) excitement or delerium, (III) relaxation or surgical anesthesia, (IV) depression or intoxication. Stage III is further divided into four planes by some anesthetists.

Stage I: The analgesia or irritation stage is characterized by tearing, mucus secretion warmth, sensation of asphyxia, peculiar and indescribable sensations and hallucinations. There may be confusion, struggle and reflex holding of the breath. There is some dulling of pain perception which becomes more intense toward the end of this stage when the patient falls asleep.

Stage II: The excitement or delerium stage is often difficult for the anesthetist to manage because there is overstimulation which may induce spasm of the larynx or pharynx. Respiratory reflexes may also be stimulated. Struggling, talking, shouting and singing are common. Vomiting, with its hazard of aspiration, may complicate matters. During the latter part of this stage the patient becomes quiet, his respirations regular and he slowly begins to relax.

Stage III: The stage of surgical anesthesia is characterized by the depression of the spinal cord and most reflexes, the corneal being the last to go. As a result, there is the complete muscular relaxation necessary for abdominal surgery. The patient is motionless, comatose, does not react to painful stimuli in any way and, under ideal conditions, respirations are deep, quiet and regular, heart rate is within safe limits and the blood pressure well above shock levels. Under these conditions vital vegetative functions are not disturbed by the surgical procedures. The further division into four planes is a highly technical matter which can be appreciated only by those with actual experience in anesthesia.

Stage IV: The stage of depression or intoxication is characterized by depression of the medullary centers, sometimes with respiratory paralysis, circulatory collapse, shock and death. It is to be
avoided at all costs even if it requires prohibition or termination
of the operation.

For this reason the anesthetist is, in a sense, in command; it is
up to him to make the decision when the patient's state of anesthesia and physical condition warrant the continuation or the termination of the operation. For these reasons too, the anesthetist
watches respiratory and cardiovascular function carefully throughout the operation.

Recovery from general anesthesia usually develops in approximately the reverse order of its development. Often there is a stage
of excitement which is a source of difficulty in management and of
danger to the patient, for he may injure himself. This must be
watched for, and in the recovery room precautions are usually taken
to protect the patient.

The depth of anesthesia required is determined by two effects:
(1) induction of sleep and (2) relaxation of muscles. In cases in
which muscular relaxation is not required, as, for example in an
operation on a limb, only sleep or unconsciousness is needed. In
the case of surgery in the abdomen, however, relaxation of the
abdominal muscles also is necessary, hence a much deeper stage
of anesthesia, one well beyond the relief of pain, is needed to induce
the abdominal relaxation which abdominal surgery requires.

As already mentioned, the dangers of anesthesia arise from the
fact that it represents a profound degree of intoxication of the
brain. This may lead to serious depression of vital functions, the
most serious of which are cardiac or respiratory depression. Some
anesthetics are more prone to induce such effects than others, and
the anesthetist and surgeon, considering both the medical and surgical status of the patient, choose the anesthetic best suited for him.
Another danger present with some types of gas anesthesia, notably
nitrous oxide used for induction, is that oxygen intake is markedly
reduced and susceptible patients, as a consequence, may suffer
serious and sometimes permanent damage to the brain.

Gas anesthetics, especially ether, leave the patient with some
discomforts due to the anesthetic. Although the newer gases tend to

ACTION OF LOCAL ANESTHESIA (PROCAINE)

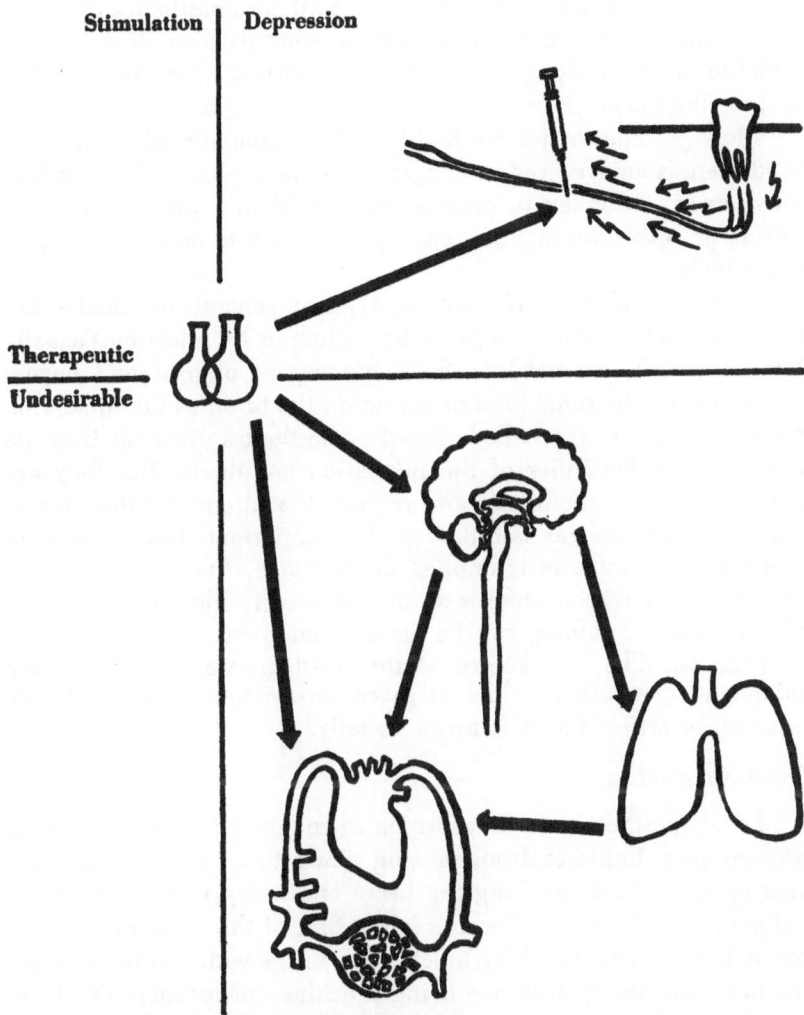

Fig. 2—Local anesthetics produce their therapeutic effects by blocking the transmission of pain impulses to the brain. Toxic effects consist of depression of the central nervous system, cardiovascular system and respiration.

be less disagreeable for the patient, many of them have special dangers of their own. It may be stated categorically at this time that in general, ether is still the safest of all gas anesthetics and may be the gas of choice in cases with serious cardiac disease. The toxicities of the newer gases are not so important in healthy patients undergoing surgery.

Most gas anesthetics are highly inflammable and when they are used there is an everpresent danger of fire or explosion. Precautions must always be taken to prevent such accidents; when they occur during an operation they are usually fatal both to patient and operating team.

Fixed anesthetics: The second type of general anesthetics are fixed anesthetics. They are given by rectum or by injection (usually intravenously) and produce the same degree of profound unconsciousness by the same kind of action on the brain as the inhalation anesthetic. They are called "fixed" anesthetics because they do not have the flexibility of the inhalation anesthetic. But they are much simpler to administer and require less attention after administration than the gas anesthetics. The important disadvantage of this type of anesthesia is implied in the name. Anesthesia is *fixed*, and if for any reason there is an urgent need to diminish the depth of drug action, nothing can be done about it except to wait for it to wear off. The best known of the fixed general anesthetics are thiopental (pentothal) which is given intravenously and tribromo-ethanol (avertin) which is given rectally.

Local Anesthetics

Local anesthetics are drugs which when applied directly to nerves prevent pain impulses from passing along these nerves, thus preventing them from reaching the brain and being registered on the patient's consciousness. Cocaine is the first of the local anesthetics, but it has been replaced by much safer drugs with similar actions, the most commonly used one being procaine (novocain). The local anesthetic may be applied as (1) an *infiltration* at the site of an incision, so that it affects the terminations of the nerves in the infiltrated area, (2) a *blocking agent* injected somewhere along the trunk of the nerve, but some distance from the site of an incision and (3) in the form of *spinal anesthesia* injected around the level of the spinal cord which serves the area of operation. These types of anesthesia also paralyze motor function in the areas involved. Finally there is (4) *surface* anesthesia in which an anesthetic which is absorbed from the skin or mucous membranes if applied to such surfaces. In this case moderate pain or itching may be relieved. Motor function is never paralyzed. Ethyl aminobenzoate (benzocaine) is one of the commonly used surface anesthetics.

In all of these three technics for local anesthesia the patient is entirely conscious and knows what is going on, because his brain has in no way been affected by the anesthetic. One of the dangers with spinal anesthesia is that the action on the spinal cord may produce considerable depression in blood pressure, an effect which should be considered with patients who are in or approaching vasomotor collapse.

In order to maintain blood pressure ephedrine or other sympathomimetic drugs are often used during the course of spinal anesthesia. Another precaution with spinal anesthesia is that it may not be administered for operations on high levels in the body, because of the danger of paralyzing vital centers in the medulla of the brain.

When spinal anesthesia is administered successfully, there is not only the advantage of its convenience for the anesthetist but also complete relaxation of the abdominal muscles which facilitates surgery in that area. The aftermath of spinal anesthesia may be prolonged headache unless precautions against this are observed. Mainly because of the good muscular relaxation, there are many surgeons who prefer to operate under this type of anesthesia whenever it is possible.

Surface anesthesia: This type of local anesthesia is induced by drugs which are absorbed from the surface of the skin and mucous membranes. Such a drug action is used mainly to relieve superficial distress (pain, itching, etc.) in skin disturbances, hemorrhoids, sore throats, and similar conditions. Ethylaminobenzoate (benzocaine, anesthesin) and tetracaine (pontocaine) are among the more commonly used drugs in this group.

It is to be noted that procaine is not absorbed from the surface of the skin and mucous membranes and that it therefore has no surface analgetic action. Cocaine is the first and one of the most potent surface anesthetics. It is rapidly absorbed from mucous membrane surfaces and is sometimes used to relieve severe pain. It is used only in very special cases, however, becaue it is a very toxic agent, and if there is a cut or abrasion on the surface anesthetized by it, absorption may be so rapid as to produce dangerous toxic effects.

Adjuvants to Anesthesia

Atropine is often used together with inhalation anesthesia to suppress excessive mucous secretions in the trachea which may interfere with respiration. The drug, incidentally, stimulates the respiratory center which is also considered advantageous.

Morphine is sometimes given as a form of premedication to allay fears and thus to enable the patient to take the anesthetic with less anxiety. On the other hand, morphine tends to depress respiration and overdosage must be avoided.

Curare (or similar drugs) is often given together with inhalation anesthesia to induce good relaxation of abdominal muscles through its paralyzing action. This effect reduces the amount of anesthesia necessary in the operation because the anesthesia merely induces the sleep while the relaxation of the abdominal muscles sufficient to permit abdominal surgery comes from the curare. The dose of curare necessary to induce such muscular relaxation usually also paralyzes the diaphragm and artificial respiration often has to be given throughout the course of curare action.

Analgesia

There are two kinds of analgesic drugs, the addictive, and the nonaddictive analgesics.

Addictive Analgesics

The narcotics are drugs which can provide a high order of relief for pain of the severest type although they must be given in a larger than ordinary dose to induce coma. In the usual therapeutic doses most of these drugs produce some degree of euphoria (a sense of well being) or elation, sluggishness or dulling of thinking, sleepiness and even behavior disturbances. In general these drugs tend to alter the patient's mental reaction to life in general as well as to pain so that he does not mind its presence even when pain does

ACTION OF MORPHINE

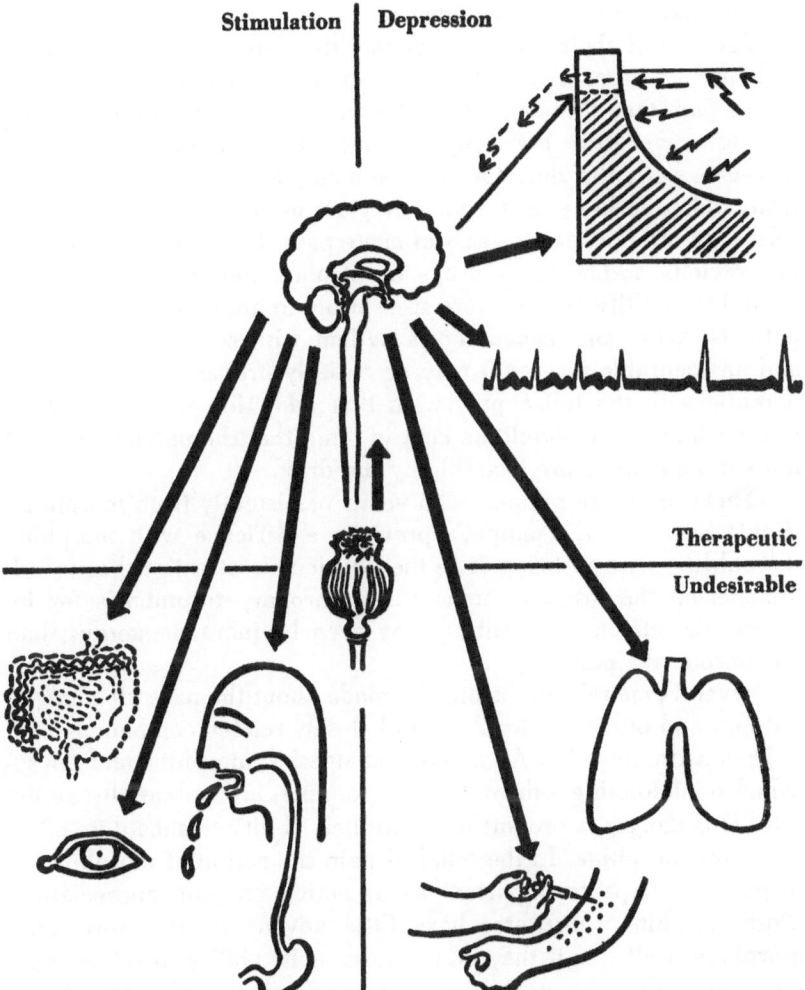

Fig. 3—Morphine has important stimulant as well as depressant actions. The major therapeutic action derives from depression of pain appreciation (elevation of pain threshold). It also slows the heart. Important undesirable effects consist of the danger of addiction, depression of respiration, constriction of the pupil, vomiting and spasm of the intestine.

not disappear. In overdosage these drugs not only produce coma but they may also cause serious depression of respiration and death. Too frequent use induces addiction.

Because of their inherent dangers the narcotics are to be used with utmost care. In situations in which the patient's reaction to severe pain may threaten his life these may be lifesaving drugs, but they are never to be given lightly. Since the likelihood of addiction increases with the duration of treatment, there is serious danger from addiction in cases in which they are used for chronic pain and relatively little danger in cases of acute pain. Patients with a history of previous addiction to drugs or alcohol, and even those with mental instability are far more susceptible to addiction than normal patients. When one encounters a patient with severe chronic pain and an incurable disease it may be entirely proper to administer a narcotic with the full appreciation that addiction will result. In a case such as this it should be kept in mind that the patient's limited life will be made more bearable by the drug.

There are some patients who vomit persistently from morphine; if this has been the patient's previous experience with morphine it would be wise to bring it to the physician's attention before administering the drug. In some cases, coronary thrombosis for instance, the effects of vomiting may even be more dangerous than the unrelieved pain.

Several generalizations may be made about the narcotic analgesics, new and old: (1) Morphine and closely related compounds tend to be constipating. (2) All narcotic analgesics, morphine and the so-called nonaddicting substitutes for example, are potentially addictive. This danger is proportionate to their ability to substitute effectively for morphine. In the relief of pain the action of morphine on mood is perhaps as important as its action on pain appreciation. Most morphine substitutes have little advantage, therefore, over morphine itself, for if they do not possess its ability to relieve anxiety and to alter mood, they are not as effective as morphine in relieving all types of severe pain. (3) It usually requires about a week or two of ordinary therapeutic dosage to induce addiction in a normal person with morphine or other addictive drugs. (4) The commonly used prescriptions (cough mixtures and antidiarrhea mixtures) which contain small amounts of morphine, present a small but everpresent addiction danger. (5) The history of morphine substitutes shows that each is introduced with a claim for nonaddiction, a claim which never is supported by the experiences which accumulate with the use of the drug. (6) Overdosage by morphine and many of its so-called substitutes may cause serious respiratory depression.

Addiction

As we have already seen, the problem of addiction goes hand in hand with the discussion of narcotic analgesic drugs. It is a problem of special importance in relation to nursing care, for the nurse may be the first to appreciate its development—a development which can seriously complicate all nursing procedures. Addiction may be simply defined as a state in which the patient's desire for a drug reaches a point at which it becomes a compelling force in his life often to the detriment of other, ordinarily important and vital drives. It is usually associated with the development of tolerance so that the addict requires and demands increasingly larger doses. The development of tolerance should furnish a clue to the beginning of addiction.

Other definitions of addiction may be found. According to a so-called pharmacologic definition, addiction depends on the development of tolerance and on the symptoms which follow withdrawal. While these symptoms are usually present in addiction as defined here, they are not always present in patients to whom the taking of drugs constitutes their most important drive. From the point of view of the social problems involved, the present tendency is to take the liberal view regardless of withdrawal symptoms, and consider a patient addicted to a drug if taking it becomes one of the most important drives in his life. This is a more practical view than the one which attempts to distinguish between habituation, dependence and addiction.

When a drug is abruptly withdrawn from an addict the withdrawal symptoms which may develop are sometimes serious enough to threaten the patient's life. Often considerable violence, nervousness, restlessness, anxiety, nausea, vomiting, sweating, weakness, convulsions and collapse may develop.

The narcotic analgesics form the most important group of addictive drugs, but by the broad definition given above, they are not the only addicting drugs. Chief among the others are the sedative drugs, the barbiturates and chloral hydrate. Alcoholism and drug addiction are in many respects similar psychologic processes. Addiction to *Cannabis indica* (marijuana, hashish, etc.) and to cocaine rarely develop as the result of therapy because they have little use in modern medicine. It is well to remember that although the Harrison Narcotic Laws serve as a protection against addiction and the acquisition of drugs by addicts, there are many drugs, which by the liberal definition, are addictive and which do not fall under the Harrison Law. Changes have been made recently to close these gaps in drug control.

Treatment of Addiction

The treatment of addiction to narcotic drugs presents one of the most serious and troublesome of all nursing problems. The cure of addiction is not always possible. It is considerably simpler, however, in the patient accidentally addicted during a painful illness than in the patient who has acquired the habit through his own devices. It is usually quite difficult to cure the latter because the addiction is often the result of neurotic difficulties which led the patient to drugs as an avenue of escape. In such a case a permanent cure is more likely when it is associated with psychotherapy. In the case of accidental addiction, as might occur in a patient with prolonged severe pain, the cure of addiction often becomes a simple matter when the illness is cured and the pain disappears, but until then is quite resistive to treatment. Thus, in any case, the cause of the addiction should be removed if a good result from treatment is to be expected.

The problems of the nurse who handles the patient being "cured" of the drug habit are very great. Patients both fear and resist treatment and withdrawal greatly, and often use the cleverest devices to obtain the drugs they are being weaned away from. There are, in general, two methods of cure: one in which the drug is abruptly withdrawn, the other in which the weaning is gradual. Wherever permitted by the health of the patient, the more quickly the drug can be withdrawn the more easily the cure can be accomplished. Often during the withdrawal period other potent drugs may be necessary to relieve the patient from the difficulties of withdrawal. While the various addicting drugs offer somewhat different problems in curing patients from the habit, the general problem is more or less the same in all cases. This is generally so because the psychologic features of the patients tend to be similar. It must be remembered that a medical cure in no way insures against the patient's returning to the drug habit promptly after release from the hospital.

Nonaddictive Analgesics

The non-narcotic analgesics are a group of drugs often used to relieve many of the common types of mild and nontraumatic pain. They are given for such things as headaches, muscle and joint pains, discomforts of colds and grippes and menstrual cramps. Since they exert virtually no effect on mental acuity and behavior—do not produce euphoria, stupor or sleepiness—they may be taken with complete safety by a patient who has to drive a car or follow some skilled or even dangerous occupation. Another characteristic of drugs in this group is their ability to reduce abnormally high temperatures, the property of antipyresis which is discussed elsewhere (page 128). For these reasons and since toxic reactions (except for allergies) are relatively rare, these drugs are frequently prescribed by the physician and bought by the layman without the physician's advice.

The best known of the analgesic is aspirin (acetylsalicylic acid), a drug belonging to a large chemical family of salicylates, all of which have essentially the same properties. Other drugs like acetophenetidin (phenacetin) and acetanilid are less frequently used since methemoglobinemia, a blood pigment disturbance, has been associated with their chronic use.

Combinations of these drugs, sometimes with caffeine, are frequently used and widely sold to the lay public through national advertising (anacin, B-C, etc.). The very common APC capsule or tablet of the hospital formulary is also one of these. There is little evidence that these common combinations are any more effective than any one of the analgesic ingredients used alone in proper dosage. There is no harm in these combinations except the increased likelihood of allergic reaction. On the other hand, combinations of these drugs with barbiturates present a special problem. The barbiturate is added to the analgesic, presumably to alter mood and assist in pain relief. Such a fixed combination implies that a fixed relationship exists between the need for each of the two effects of the two drugs in the treatment of pain in all cases. This is far from the truth, some patients requiring more drug for pain relief (the analgesic) and some more for mood effect (the barbiturate). When attempting to increase the dose, to intensify one of these two effects with a fixed combination, the dose of the other drug is automatically increased. In some instances this may result in overdosage of one or the other drug. Since there is no need to put each drug in the same capsule, the two may be taken separately as needed without the danger just described.

In the history of the development of analgesic drugs there have been some experiences with dangerous drug reactions which may be mentioned here with value. Aminopyrine (pyramidon) was, at one time, one of the most popular members of the group because of its dependability. During the past twenty years its use has been largely discontinued because of disasters caused by it. As the drug gained in popularity years ago, a serious blood dyscrasia, angranulocytosis, made its appearance and increased in incidence. Only after a surprisingly large number of deaths were the drug and disease connected. It was proved that in sensitive patients aminopyrine could, even in very small dosage, cause this fatal disease. A similar history is obtained in the case of cinchophen (atophan and neo-atophan). Here the use of this effective analgesic was associated with a rise in the incidence of another fatal disease, acute yellow atrophy of the liver.

The analgesic drugs which are used widely today (salicylates, acetanilid, and acetophenetidin) rarely cause serious toxic reactions and, in general, they may be used relatively freely and without grave danger. In the event of new analgesic drugs, however, the history of aminopyrine and cinchophen should be borne in mind until the safety of the new drug is proven; a dangerous toxic reaction is hardly justified in the case of a medicament for the relief of a simple headache.

Specific Analgesia

The most desirable approach to the problem of pain relief is specific analgesia which acts on the physiologic or pathologic mechanism which causes the pain. Unfortunately, however, it is not often a practical approach. Well established examples of such relief are the action of nitroglycerin in an attack of angina pectoris, gynergen in an attack of migraine headache and calcium in an attack of lead colic. In the case of the anginal attack, the pain is caused by a spasm of the coronary arteries, the nitroglycerin acts directly on the cause of pain by relaxing the arteries, thus relieving pain by correcting a physiologic disturbance. The action of nitroglycerin does not involve the nervous system at all in its mechanism of relief and differs, therefore, from the action of drugs on the brain to dull pain perception. In the case of nitroglycerin, the pain mechanism is no longer present; in the case of the drug acting on the nervous system, the pain mechanism may well be present, it is only that the patient does not appreciate it. Such examples of specific pain relief will not be discussed further here, but will be considered in the sections in which they properly belong, namely the physiologic systems in which they operate.

Psychologic Disturbances

Depressant Drugs

One group of drugs used in psychologic disturbances are the depressants; they are most commonly given for nervousness, excitement, hysteria and insomnia.

Nervousness

One of the common complaints in life in general as well as in medicine is nervousness. The patient suffers from anxiety about incidents and events which do not merit such intense concern, or he may have anxiety about events which have not occurred. The anxiety may disturb him to the extent that he cannot perform his duties efficiently or at all, that he makes serious errors in judgment. He may not be able to sleep to the extent that he is always fatigued. The internal commotion may seriously interfere with his vegetative functions. Some patients have real complaints due to organic disease, but the concern they suffer over the possibilities of the illness may cause more trouble than the illness itself. For these reasons it may be desirable to relieve the patient of his nervousness or anxieties regardless of whether he has organic disease. It must be borne in mind that such symptomatic relief is never a cure or a substitute for adequate psychotherapy in cases which require it. On the other hand, the temporary rest and relief may permit the patient to adjust better to his anxieties, so that he can later do without medication. If his anxieties are over an actual illness, he may, after recovery, find that sedative medication is unnecessary.

The drugs to be used in such situations require careful consideration, for although the original intention may be to use a sedative drug for a limited period of time, such unstable personalities as those which require sedatives may attach themselves firmly to the drug and resist giving up the acquired support provided by the drug. It is often wiser, therefore, to attempt to relieve anxieties by reassurance that the patient's difficulties are under control, that they do not merit anxieties and that every eventuality has been provided for. Usually such reassurance given by doctor or nurse has only short-lived effectiveness. In some highly suggestive patients, any medication, regardless of its action—even a completely inert placebo—will for a limited time at least, provide good relief from anxieties. As mentioned elsewhere (page 7) such a procedure is fully justified, provided the patient is not given the impression that doctor and nurse are playing a game with him, that necessary and effective specific medication is being withheld and that harmful substitution for an effective drug is being made. Other patients are resistive to purely suggestive therapy of any type and require fairly potent drugs to alleviate their anxieties.

Sedation: The drugs used to relieve anxieties and to ease tension states are usually called sedatives. In general, all drugs which perform such a function tend to be habituating drugs, and this, together with the personality which requires such a drug action, makes the danger of habituation a formidable one if the drug is continued for any length of time. In addition, other toxic symptoms may also develop. In the case of the barbiturate drugs, after taking them for an extended period, sudden cessation may be followed by convulsions. It is a serious matter, therefore, to embark on a program of drug sedation for a period of any length, and the dangers involved should be carefully weighed.

There are many drugs which may be used for purposes of sedation: in general they are the same drugs that are used for insomnia and excitement. The material most frequently taken for this purpose by the layman himself is alcohol. Alcoholic beverages tend to allay fears and anxieties and have much the same type of action on the brain as the common sedative tablet. This, of course, accounts for a large measure of the widespread use of alcohol. The danger of habituation to such a drug action is well exemplified by the large number of alcoholics.

The commonest drugs prescribed by the medical profession are the barbiturates. In addition there are the bromides, urethane derivatives and a continual flow of new sedative drugs. So many of these are available that it is not possible for any one to have a large experience with all of them. Most physicians tend to depend on only a few drugs of this series and to concentrate their experience on them. This is the wisest course, not because any one of them has proved superiority over the others, but because experience with any drug improves the results one obtains with it. The barbiturate series constitutes a long list of drugs, the most frequently used of which are perhaps phenobarbital and pentobarbital (nembutal). There is no doubt that new sedatives will continue to be introduced by drug manufacturers. Any claims for superiority are to be critically considered, for the experience with the large number already on hand, each originally introduced with the same enthusiasm, has proved that few superiority claims ever survive trial. The choice of a barbiturate is better made on the basis of speed and duration of action rather than any other qualities claimed, for there is little difference in the quality of sedation itself.

It is well to note that in many instances in which so-called sedative doses of barbiturate drugs are prescribed, the doses are too small to exert a pharmacologic effect and, therefore, act solely through suggestion much as a placebo. In many instances, an effective sedative action cannot be obtained with these drugs until an observable effect on the mental acuity of the patient is also obtained. These effects might be drowsiness, dullness, or a state closely akin to the early stages of alcohol action, an action not desirable in a man working at a skilled or dangerous occupation, but not of such importance in the hospitalized patient.

Excitement

Excitement may be an intensified state of nervousness. Sometimes, however, it may progress into a state of *mania* which is dangerous to the patient and to those near him. In such states the degree of sedation induced has to be intense enough to produce behavior changes in the patient, sometimes to the extent of anesthetization. Such a situation often arises either after an alcoholic spree or in psychotic patients. In such instances the patient may have to be restrained and the drug given by injection. Clearly only potent drugs are effective in such cases. In many instances, however, larger doses of the frequently used barbiturate drugs will serve.

Hysteria

The hysterical state may closely resemble the excitement state in the patient's violence of action, although in this situation usually the only one in danger is the patient himself. Here, too, the situation may urgently demand an intense degree of drug action.

Insomnia

Insomnia is, in most instances, an expression of a tension state. The same problems exist as in the case of simple nervousness. In insomnia the patient spends much time and effort in trying to induce or to force himself to sleep, and as a consequence he may be more fatigued when he arises in the morning than when he went to bed. The use of drugs in chronic insomnia presents the same dangers in their continued use as in nervousness, and the same caution must be given to their application. Although it is easy to put a patient to sleep with a drug it does not provide a solution to the insomnia problem.

There are some devices not requiring drugs which may be of help in insomnia. A hot or cold shower, a midnight snack, a glass of beer or ale, or something stronger, may be tried before retiring. Often, unfortunately, it will be discovered that the patient has already exhausted these possibilities himself, and they are presently ineffective.

Before a drug is given to the patient the type of insomnia should be defined. Two kinds may broadly be considered: the one in which the patient has difficulty in falling asleep, but once asleep sleeps well, and the one in which the patient falls asleep easily but awakens in the early morning and cannot fall asleep again. The drug which produces its effects quickly would be more suited for the first instance while the drug which produces its effects slowly and persistently would be the better drug for the second type. For this reason it is well to explore the nature of the insomnia as well as the speed and duration of action of drugs which are to be given for insomnia. Practical differences in curves of action are to be found among the barbiturate drugs, phenobarbital being a slow-acting one and pentobarbital the one with a rapid curve of action. An especially important hazard for some patients, especially those who work at highly skilled and dangerous occupations, is the so-called "hangover" after the long-acting drugs. This may be even more disastrous than the fatigue from not sleeping. In each case the drug used will have to be fitted to the patient's type of insomnia and his response to drugs.

Convulsions

Convulsions are purposeless movements of the extremities and the body, sometimes violent in nature, and sometimes a matter of great danger to the patient. In some cases there may be only one episode, as in poisonings; in other cases, the chronic epileptic for instance, they occur repeatedly. Convulsions are the result of some kind of irritation to the brain, low calcium level in the blood, brain tumor, increased intra-cranial pressure, strychnine poisoning, drug actions and intoxications of various types. Convulsions are common in infants as well as in adults. In some psychologic conditions and in some intoxications they are deliberately induced with drugs. During convulsions a patient may injure himself seriously unless the nurse on the scene takes the proper precautions.

Anticonvulsant drugs may be of two types (1) the general depressant, and (2) the specific anticonvulsant. The general depressants include the anesthetics, large doses of barbiturates, paraldehyde and similar drugs. The specific anticonvulsants have less diffuse depressant action and may be taken without producing sleepiness or stupor. There is a special case for phenobarbital, a barbiturate which appears to exert a specific action against epileptic convulsions not present in other barbiturates, preventing them in doses which do not produce somnolence. In addition, the slight depressant action which phenobarbital may exert may be helpful, for in the case of chronic deteriorated epileptics their behavior with phenobarbital is sometimes more tolerable than when they are given specific anticonvulsant drugs, which do not have a sedative action.

Epilepsy is really the only important disease in which the specific anticonvulsant drugs have an important use. For this condition there are several types of drugs available, the choice depending largely on the precise nature of the epileptic disturbance, whether it be grand mal, petit mal, or the psychomotor equivalent. In convulsions due to other causes, either the cause has to be removed or counteracted or a general anesthetic has to be administered. In some cases dilantin, the anti-epileptic drug may be useful. When general anesthesia is used to suppress convulsions, the greatest of care is required to suppress the convulsion without depressing vital functions at the same time.

Stimulants

Stimulation of the central nervous system is used (1) to arouse patients from a state of depression, stupor, or coma; (2) to increase reflex activity in cases of depressed respiration or circulation due to disease, shock or drug intoxication; (3) to induce convulsions in the treatment of psychologic disorders. Drugs which act directly on the vital centers of the brain are the ones used today although strychnine, a drug which acted principally on the spinal cord, was often used years ago. The modern convulsive or analeptic drugs may act on the cerebrum, the cerebellum, or on the vital centers, the respiratory or the vasomotor centers. There are also drugs which have highly specific central actions, such as apomorphine, a drug which stimulates the vomiting center in the brain and is used to empty the stomach in cases of poisoning. These special cases, however, will be considered in other sections.

Some patients in a state of mental depression of psychologic origin, as a hangover from drinking, overwork or lack of sleep, may be temporarily helped by the use of mildly stimulant or cephalotropic drugs such as amphetamine (benzedrine) and related drugs. These drugs may also contribute a sense of well being; in addition, they seem to decrease the appetite in instances in which obesity is due to psychogenic overeating. When used regularly, dependence may develop to such stimulants and this is seriously to be considered. There is also the fact that such stimulation may permit patients with heart disease or other serious ailments to work at times when their normal fatigue would prevent them from overexerting themselves.

Finally, stimulants are used with profoundly depressed patients who must be aroused to witness, or sign a document, a will perhaps. Often such temporary stimulation can be brought about despite profound depression. Such drug awakenings have legal overtones which we cannot argue here.

In serious diseases, such as shock and drug intoxication, respiration, circulation and the patient's reflex activity may be profoundly depressed, sometimes to the extent that his life is seriously endangered. To some extent this can be counteracted by the administration of oxygen and artificial respiration, and the use of blood or blood substitutes. For immediate effects, however, a rapidly acting drug may be a life-saving measure. The drugs often used in these cases are the so-called analeptics, nikethamide (coramine), epinephrine and related compounds. In cases in which the heart has stopped the drug must be injected directly into the heart. In many instances such a treatment may start respirations going, make the heart beat, elevate the blood pressure or bring about reflex nervous activity. In many of these cases the effect may last only a few instants, after which the patient's condition deteriorates rapidly. In other cases the brief stimulation may start things going in the right direction and the properly regulated use of these drugs may save the patient's life. To be effective these drugs require constant vigilance.

The special use of picrotoxin or other analeptic drugs in the treatment of barbiturate poisoning also deserves mention. In this case the analeptics are used continuously over the period of profound depression to induce a near-convulsive state. This treatment continues until the patient's reflex activity returns.

Psychoses

The psychoses form one of the most serious problems in all

medicine. The psychotics are a group of chronic patients who are not only useless but may be dangerous; their large number constitutes a heavy drain on our economic and social structure. There are more psychotic patients in hospitals than for all other illnesses put together. Until relatively recently there was no effective treatment for these disturbed people, but with the advent of convulsion therapy about twenty years ago hope appeared for many. In some instances this kind of therapy has produced permanent alleviation of symptoms; in other cases the apparent cure has been temporary; and in still others, while the restoration of mental health has never been complete, it has been sufficient to permit the patients to return to their homes and function to a limited extent in a normal social environment.

The drugs that produce the necessary convulsions, insulin and pentylenetetrazol (metrazol), have largely been replaced by electrical apparatus which can better control the development of convulsions. In some instances, however, drugs are still used. To avoid accidents due to the violence of convulsions, paralyzing drugs such as curare are used which prevent the thrashing of the limbs but which do not interfere with the effect of the treatment on the brain.

Tonics

In connection with drugs acting as nervous system stimulants the common request for a "general tonic" should also be discussed. Often patients will urgently demand such a medicament to "pep them up generally," "make them feel better," "more ambitious," "more efficient," "stronger and less easily fatigued." This request of drugs without a specific action on the fundamental disease problem seems like a reasonable and simple one to the patient.

The myth about the "tonic" developed in times when there was virtually no specific cure for disease, and the concoctions given had only psychogenic effects. The idea that there is a general tonic medication persists, not because we have one, but because there is a need and a desire for one. In some cases, such an effect can be temporarily produced by suggestive medication.

That such a type of drug action is desirable is beyond question, but how to obtain it is still another matter. There are drugs which can make patients feel better through a dulling action on the brain, morphine and related drugs, alcohol, the barbiturates, but these all have obvious dangers in addiction. Drugs like amphetamine (benzedrine) may exert such an effect temporarily, but not in all cases. Here, too, is a danger of drug dependence. The general principle to bear in mind is the fact that any medication given with enthusiasm and conviction may produce this action; this is probably why so many people feel better after taking vitamins. More often than not, they act through the psyche rather than through a true need for vitamins. In diagnosed disease, the properly applied specific treatment may do all the things required of a tonic, but the fact remains that in cases of undiagnosed disease or incurable disease, any tonic action obtained from a prescription is most likely due to a psychologic effect.

Organs of Special Sense

The Eye

Because the eye is such an important organ for the function of the individual, and because of its sensitivity to pain and irritants, great anxiety and much distress attends all acute eye disorders. From time to time, there are serious emergencies involving the eye in which that organ can be saved by prompt and effective action.

The eye is a spherical organ which lies in the skull and is well protected by the bony case and the eyelids. It consists of the heavy wall which forms its coat; a lens inside which divides the eye into two compartments (one in front and one in back); the retina or nerve lining which is sensitive to light and color and conducts images through the optic nerve to the brain; and the iris which opens and closes to permit more or less light to reach the retina. The outer surface of the eye is extremely sensitive to irritants and is bathed continuously with tears which form in the lacrymal glands in the upper lid and are drained through the nasolacrymal duct into the nose.

The eye may be affected by trauma, infections, inflammations and degenerative processes. These may cause pain, redness, a discharge, or may interfere with vision. We are neither concerned here with the mechanical changes in the lens of the eye which may require correction by glasses, nor with eye-muscle variations which may require exercise for correction. We are concerned, however, with the use of drugs in eye disorders.

Many drugs are applied directly to the outer surface of the eye either to produce surface effects, or to be absorbed in order to produce effects within the eye. Since the surface of the eye is so sensitive to irritants, irritation by drugs is a commonplace. In general, if irritation of the eye is to be avoided or minimized and the best results are to be obtained, the solutions applied to the eye should resemble the composition of tears as much as possible in concentration and acidity or alkalinity (i.e. isotonic and of the same pH as tears).

Particles and other foreign bodies which get into the conjunctiva may cause considerable pain. Often the irritation is worsened when the patient rubs the eye, and he presents himself with an acutely reddened eye. If the particles cannot be easily removed, bland eye washes (collyria) should be applied. If the pain continues, a local anesthetic may be applied until the foreign particle can be removed. This will prevent further damage by rubbing. Sometimes embedded particles are pushed further into the conjunctiva by careless handling, and the nurse should be wary of any but the gentlest manipulations.

Infections of the conjunctiva were formerly treated with the mildest form of local antiseptics. At one time boric acid was the drug of choice but so many serious accidents have occured through its accidental use in intravenous medications, that it has been removed from the formularies of many hospitals. Boric acid in the home, however, is not as dangerous as in the hospital because drugs in the home medical cabinet are not given parenterally. In general, however, these mild antiseptics for the eye, boric acid, silver proteinates like argyrol, zinc salts, the yellow oxides of mercury, etc., have largely been discarded for the far more effective and less irritating antibiotics.

From time to time serious damage to the eye occurs as the result of accidents with caustic materials. The scarring of the conjunctiva which may occur as the result of such an accident may lead to blindness or require an operation. The first step in such a case is immediately to wash the eye with bland fluids. If the material is known to be an acid, a mild alkali such as sodium bicarbonate should be used in the wash water; conversely if the caustic is known to be an alkali, mild acids such as vinegar should be added to the wash water. Cortisone or ACTH used promptly after eye accidents may stop the inflammatory process and save the eye.

Mydriatics and Miotics

Mydriatics and miotics are often used in examining and treating the eye. For the purpose of a thorough examination of the retina and lens, dilatation (mydriasis) of the pupil is desirable. In producing this effect, unfortunately, pressure in the eye may rise and cause acute glaucoma, a painful condition which sometimes results in blindness. This danger is greatest in those who have the beginnings of glaucoma but it is ever-present in patients over the age of 45. For this reason an examination of the eye making use of mydriatics is limited to younger patients. In instances in which it is essential to dilate the pupil in older patients special precautions are taken. Instead of using atropine or homatropine, drugs of the epinephrine series are given.

Mydriasis and the paralysis of accomodation which may accompany it often interferes with near vision, especially reading; for that reason, after the examination is over, the oculist may administer drugs to counteract the effect of the atropine. Such drugs which constrict the pupil are called *miotics*. In addition to inducing constriction they are often used in the treatment of glaucoma to facilitate drainage and decrease the intra-ocular pressure. In general the drugs which are used to constrict the pupil belong to the cholinergic or parasympathomimetic group of autonomic drugs, and the drugs used to dilate the pupil belong to the parasympatholytic or sympathomimetic drugs. These are discussed in more detail in the section on autonomic drugs (page 115.)

The Ear

The ear is concerned with two functions, the sense of hearing and the sense of balance. These may be considered separately, for although there is only one nerve, it is divided, each part going to one of two separate organs. These organs, one for hearing and one for vestibular sense (or balance) are distinct and otherwise unrelated.

Disturbances in hearing are either congenital or acquired; they arise from infections, degenerative disease or injury. Except for the occasional use of a specific drug in infections, treatment is usually physical or surgical. Occasionally ear drops are placed in the ear canal to ease pain or act on local infections.

Disturbances in vestibular function, characterized by dizziness, arise in many conditions. They may seriously interfere with walking and in maintaining an erect posture in general. In addition to disease, disturbances in vestibular function may arise because of sudden postural changes such as occur in travel, especially aboard ship or in an airplane. Intoxication may cause vestibular disease. Often vestibular disturbances persist for a long period of time with partial, if not total, disability.

There are many forms of treatment for vestibular disease none of which is consistently effective. Dehydration together with strict limitation of salt intake is a popular form of therapy at present. Recently, antihistaminic drugs, such as dimenhydrinate (dramamine), have been used but these drugs do not live up to their original promise in all instances.

Autonomic Nervous System

The autonomic or vegetative nervous system, in contrast with the central nervous system, is concerned only with the automatic functions of the body, those which keep the machine working: the beating of the heart, the activity of the intestines and secretory glands, the tone of the arteries, the activity of the uterus, etc. It has no direct concern with voluntary or cerebral function and is composed of two separate, and to a large degree, antagonistic divisions. These are the sympathetic (sometimes called the lumbodorsal) system and the parasympathetic (sometimes called the vagal or bulbo-sacral) system. When we speak of systems as being antagonistic we simply state that each has an opposing effect on the organs they serve. Thus, the sympathetic accelerates the heart and the parasympathetic slows it; the parasympathetic intensifies peristaltic action in the intestine and the sympathetic relaxes it; the parasympathetic constricts the pupil and the sympathetic dilates it.

The condition or activity of each organ under the dual influence of these systems is always in balance and its precise state at any moment depends on the state of balance between the opposing forces. It depends, in other words, on which is the stronger influence. Thus the effect of one system is seen clearly only when it overwhelms the influence of the other; under normal conditions the two are about equal in tone and balance each other. Pronounced autonomic effects may be produced by two mechanisms which upset the state of balance; stimulation of one system or depression of the opposing system. Thus the pupil of the eye can be dilated by stimulation of the sympathetic nerve or the depression of the parasympathetic nerve to the pupil, each effect permitting sympathetic influence to predominate. The heart can be slowed by stimulation of the parasympathetic or depression of the sympathetic influence over the heart, each action permitting parasympathetic influence over the heart to predominate. That is to say, intensification of an effect by stimulation or by removing the opposition to it.

The functions which can be altered by such influences are diffuse, for the vegetative nervous system exerts its control over most organs and over the arterial system of the entire body. They are summarized in table 2 and figure 4.

Drugs are now available which stimulate or mimic the actions of these two nervous systems. Other drugs, also available, selectively depress or paralyze the vegetative nervous system and antagonize the drugs which mimic it. With drugs alone it is thus possible to reproduce the effects of stimulation or depression of the two autonomic nervous systems in the manner just described. They can accelerate or slow the heart, dilate or constrict the pupil, intensify or retard intestinal activity. The group of drugs which exert this type of action have been called collectively, autonomic drugs. They are not only of considerable academic interest, but some are of great importance from the practical point of view. Four categories of these drugs will be considered briefly.

Sympathomimetic or Adrenergic Drugs

The sympathomimetic or adrenergic drugs are those which, in part at least, mimic the effect of stimulation of the sympathetic nervous system. Outstanding effects are stimulation of the heart and

Table 2—Effects of Autonomic Drugs

Organ	Sympathomimetic	Parasympathomimetic
Pupil	dilated	constricted
Heart		
rate	accelerated	slowed
work	increased	decreased
Arteries	constricted	dilated
coronary	dilated	constricted
Bronchi	dilated	constricted
Gl tract		
motility	decreased	increased
secretions	decreased	increased
sphincters	contracted	relaxed
Urinary		
bladder	relaxed	contracted
Uterus (pregnant)	stimulated	stimulated
Skin	pallor	——
Sweat glands	inhibited	stimulated
Adrenal	——	stimulated
Salivary glands	inhibited	stimulated

rise in blood pressure by the constriction of most arteries. The adrenal gland normally produces a hormone, epinephrine or adrenalin, which reproduces this effect. Epinephrine, as a drug of commerce, is obtained from the adrenal glands of cattle (also synthetically). It is the prototype of all sympathomimetic drugs. As a result of its effect on the heart and blood pressure, it increases the work of the heart. One of its disagreeable attributes is that it induces anxiety and nervousness. Since epinephrine is not absorbed from the gastro-intestinal tract it must be given by injection or by inhalation of an aerosol. It is an extremely potent drug: its action develops quickly and is of short duration. As indicated, it has disadvantages which tend to limit its use to cases for which it has no substitutes and which are important enough to balance its disadvantages.

There are many drugs similar to epinephrine in chemical structure and action, differing from it usually in minor, and occasionally, in important respects. Some of them do not elevate the blood pres-

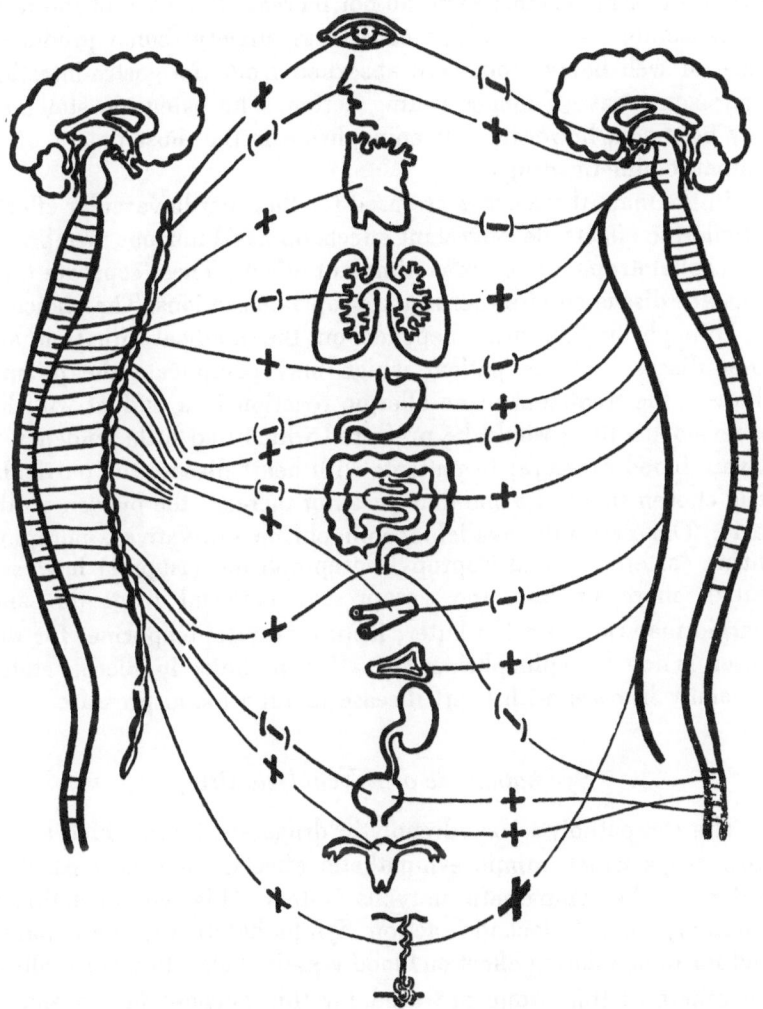

Fig. 4—Diagramatic representation of the autonomic nervous system; the sympathetic on the left, the parasympathetic on the right. Each system produces either stimulation or depression of a particular organ and, in general, each tends to oppose the other. Stimulation is indicated by a plus sign (+) and depression by a minus sign (—). The respective autonomic drugs produce similar effects.

sure to the same extent; some do not increase the work of the heart or accelerate its rate; others cause less anxiety; some produce a sense of well being; some are absorbed from the gastro-intestinal tract; some have a longer lasting action. The categoric statement may be made, however, that epinephrine is the most potent of all sympathomimetic drugs.

In the main these drugs are used for their cardiovascular effects, antiallergic effects, decongestant effects on nasal mucous membranes and cephalotropic or cerebral stimulant effects. These separate functions are discussed elsewhere in appropriate sections. The choice of an epinephrine-like drug depends on the medical situation and other diseases of the patient which may complicate the picture. Thus, in the treatment of an allergic reaction in a patient with hypertension, a drug would be preferred which had little tendency to elevate blood pressure; in patients with heart disease the particular drug chosen should be one that does not increase the burden on the heart. The presently available epinephrine derivatives, norepinephrine (arterenol) and isopropyl norepinphrine (isuprel) have separated, more or less, the vasopressor material from the antiallergic material, and the latter, isopropyl norepinephrine, for this reason is now the epinephrine derivative of choice in allergic states, especially in cases with heart disease or high blood pressure.

Sympatholytic or Adrenolytic Drugs

The sympatholytic or adrenolytic drugs are those which antagonize drugs which mimic sympathetic effects. They also paralyze or depress the sympathetic nervous system. This type of action is commonly called "blockade" action. Sympatholytic drugs are mainly used for their dilating effect on blood vessels. Tolazoline (priscoline) and others of this group are used for this purpose in vasospastic and thromboembolic disease. In addition, as explained on page 270, they are used in diagnostic tests of pheochromocytoma (tumor of adrenal gland).

Since increased arterial tone plays an important part in producing high blood pressure, it was thought that the sympatholytic drugs, by producing a type of drug sympathectomy, might be useful in the treatment of hypertension. This, unfortunately, has not yet

ACTION OF ADRENERGIC DRUGS (EPINEPHRINE)

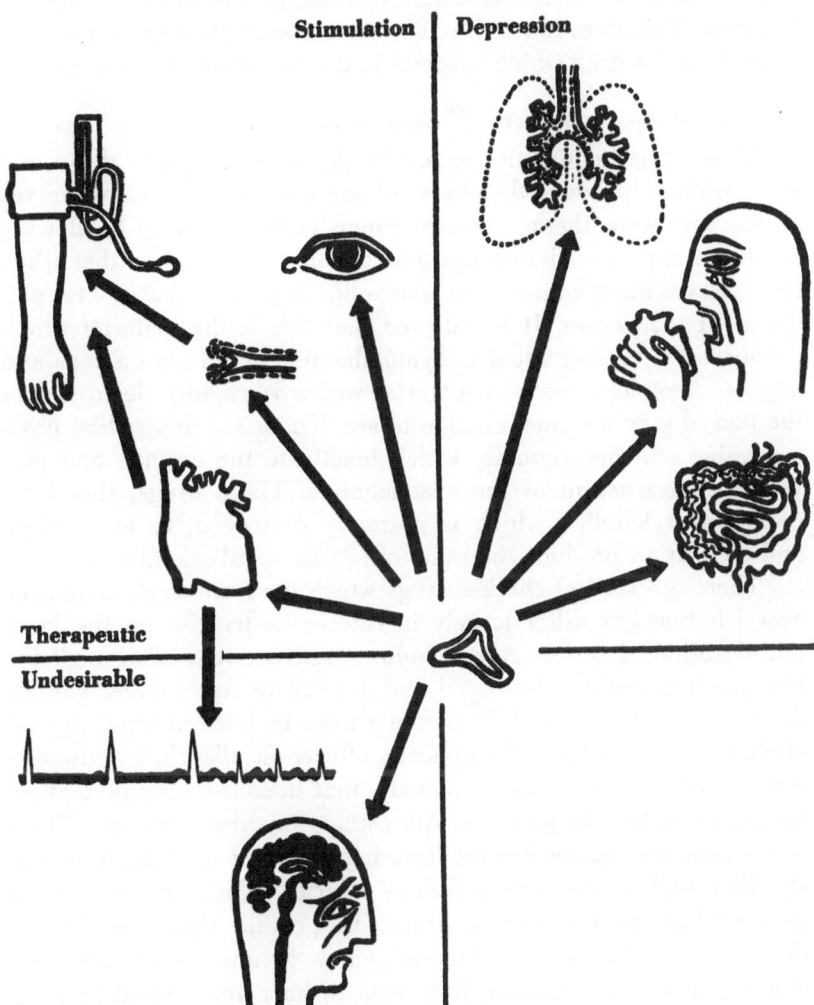

Fig. 5—The therapeutic action of the adrenergic drugs are both stimulant and depressant, the toxic effects usually arise from stimulation, producing anxiety, palpitations and sometimes marked elevation of blood pressure.

proved to be the case. Recent newspaper reports of good results from such drugs (methonium compounds) are not only premature but they also fail to describe serious toxic effects which are known to occur. This does not imply, however, that continued search may not yet yield a drug which is useful in the treatment of hypertension.

Parasympathomimetic, Vagomimetic, or Cholinergic Drugs

Parasympathomimetic, vagomimetic, or cholinergic drugs are those which reproduce the effects of stimulation of the vagus nerves or the parasympathetic nervous system (table 2), such as slowing the heart and constricting the pupils. There is evidence that when these nerves are stimulated, acetylcholine is produced at the terminations of the nerves. It is believed that this is the material which produces the typical vagal or sympathomimetic effects on cells and organs. Acetylcholine is a material which is rapidly destroyed in the body by an enzyme, cholinesterase. There are drugs, like physostigmine and neostigmine, which inactivate the enzyme and prevent the destruction of the acetylcholine. These drugs, therefore, permit acetylcholine which is normally destroyed, to accumulate and thereby to produce the same effects as vagal stimulation.

There are several choline drugs which have the same actions as acetylcholine but differ largely in rate of destruction in the body and duration of action. Acetylcholine itself is not used in medicine because it is rapidly destroyed and difficult to store. Other choline drugs, however, are used. It should always be born in mind that all cholinergic drugs have the opposite effects on allergic reactions as the sympathomimetic drugs, namely, that their use may precipitate an allergic attack in patients with asthma or other allergies. These drugs may also cause intense lowering of blood pressure and constriction of the coronary arteries—arteries which respond in an unusual way to cholinergic drugs. In general they are difficult drugs to take because of the frequency of unpleasant reactions. When one is administered, it is wise to have the patient in a recumbent position (should he faint from low blood pressure) and to keep the antidote, atropine, close at hand. The proper dose of atropine should already be in a syringe ready for prompt administration if the patient begins to complain of cardiac oppression or an allergic reaction, to vomit or show other ill effects.

ACTION OF PARASYMPATHOMIMETIC DRUGS (METHACHOLINE)

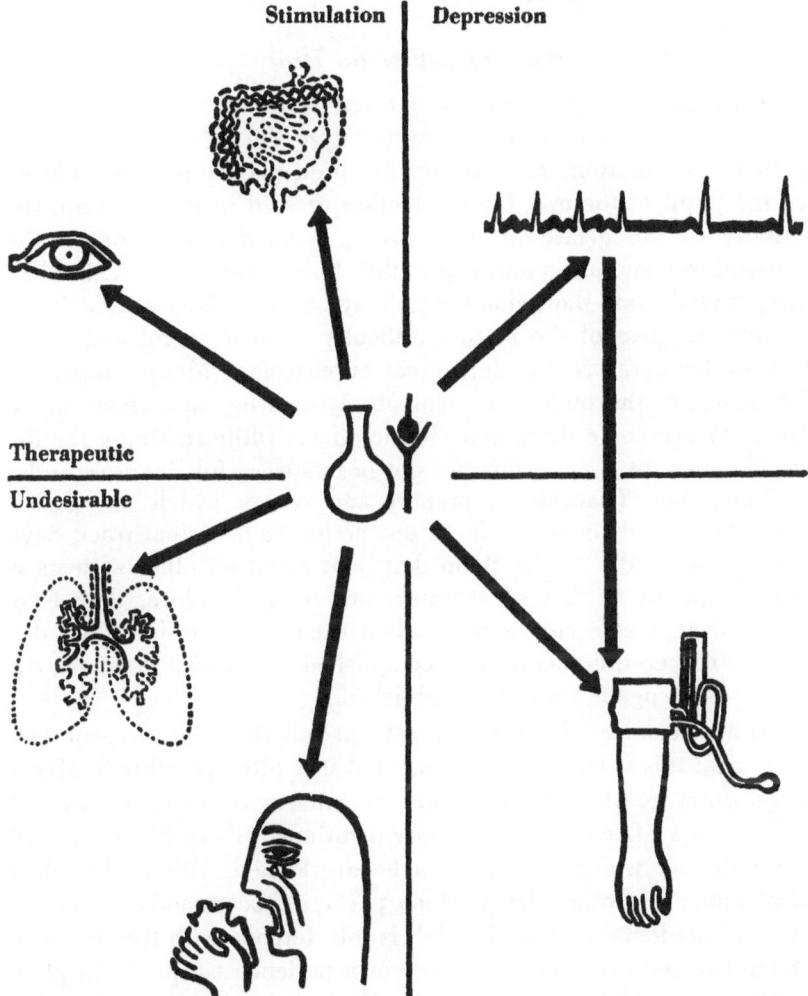

Fig. 6—The therapeutic actions of the parasympathomimetic drugs are both stimulant and depressant. The toxic effects are related to depression of blood pressure, constriction of the bronchi and induction of allergic reactions.

These drugs are used for their effects on intestinal activity, bladder activity, neuromuscular function, the pupil of the eye and in cardiac arrhythmias.

Parasympatholytic Drugs

Parasympatholytic drugs are those which are antagonistic to cholinergic drugs and depress or paralyze the effects of parasympathetic stimulation. These drugs are used mainly for their effects on the pupil of the eye, the production of acid in the stomach, the activity of the gastro-intestinal tract, mucous production in the tracheal tree and as an antidote to the cholinergic drugs. While they are generally safe their side effects may be most disagreeable. They produce dryness of the mouth, difficulty in near vision and elevation of temperature through sweat suppression. Many substitutes for atropine, the major parasympatholytic drug, have been introduced to overcome these undesirable effects while retaining the desirable ones. In general this has not been successful. More recently, methantheline (banthine), prantyl and others which are potent blockaders of cholinergic effects on the gastro-intestinal tract, have been introduced with the claim that their effect on other systems is not as intense as that of atropine and that, therefore, they have fewer disagreeable side actions when used in gastro-intestinal disease. Whether this has been accomplished to an important degree with these drugs is yet to be established.

It has been stated that the parasympatholytic drugs are generally safe ones; this is true to the extent that it is often possible to give a large dose, producing symptoms of intense discomfort, without serious after effects. But as already mentioned, there is one area of grave danger which should never be overlooked. This is the effect of atropine and other drugs which paralyze accommodation in the eye, an incidental action of which is interference with the drainage of fluid in the eye. Such an effect in a patient susceptible to glaucoma may precipitate an acute attack of glaucoma. It appears that this complication is more likely to result from the direct application to the eye than when given systemically.

ACTION OF PARASYMPATHOLYTIC DRUGS (ATROPINE)

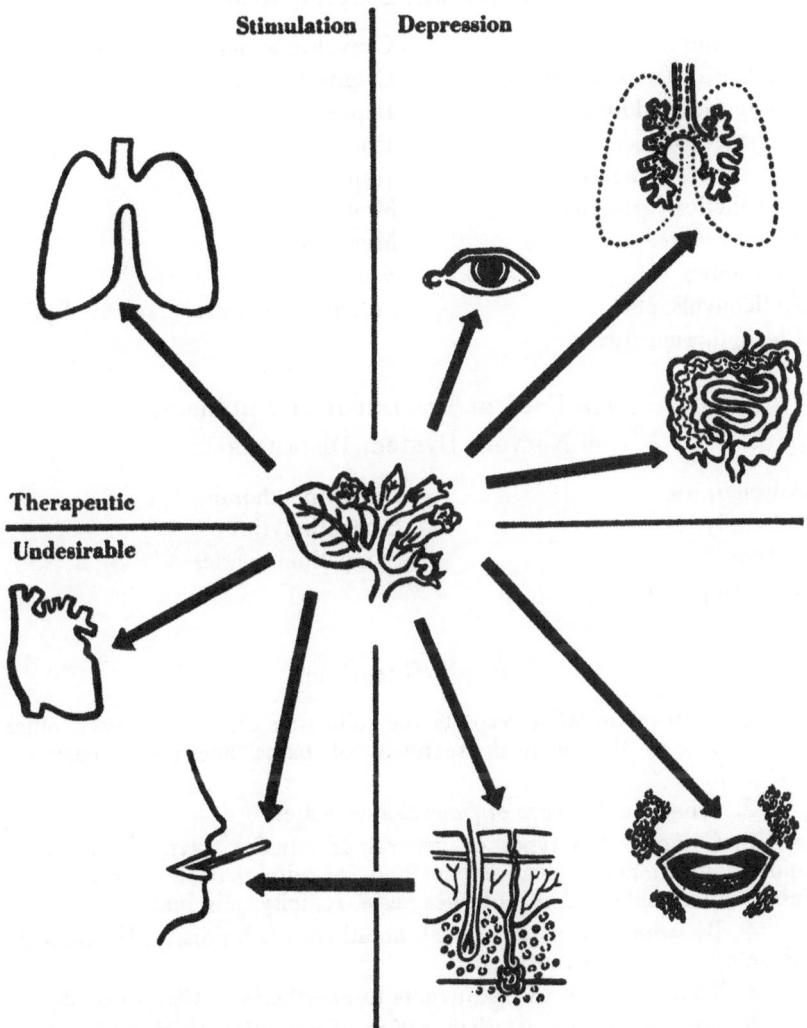

Fig. 7—The therapeutic actions of the parasympatholytic drugs stimulate respiration, depress bronchial secretion, bronchial spasm and intestinal spasm. The toxic effects slow the heart, suppress salivation and sweating and raise the temperature.

Drugs Used in Treatment of
Central Nervous System Disorders

Analeptics

Analgesics (nonaddictive)

Analgesics (addictive)

Anesthetics (local)

Anesthetics (surface)

Anesthetics (general)

Anodynes, see Analgesics

Antibiotics

Anticonvulsants

Chemotherapeutics

Convulsants, see Analeptics

Counterirritants

Depressants

Hormones

Hypnotics

Miotics

Mydriatics

Sedatives.

Stimulants (central), see Analeptics

Drugs Used in Treatment of Autonomic
Nervous System Disorders

Adrenergics

Adrenolytics

Autonomics

Parasympatholytics

Parasympathomimetics

Sympatholytics

Sympathomimetics

Study Questions

1. Indicate in what respects the following differ from each other in relation to the medical treatment of pain: anesthesia, narcosis, analgesia.

2. What are the types of general anesthetics?

3. Compare the types of general anesthetics, giving advantages and disadvantages as regards: methods of administration, ease of administration, safety, depth of anesthesia, toxicity, elimination.

4. By what means are local anesthetics administered? Indicate advantages and disadvantages.

5. What is meant by "adjuvants to anesthesia"? Give examples.

6. What is the characteristic action of narcotics which makes them especially useful in the relief of pain?

7. In what way does this characteristic become a special hazard in the use of such drugs?

8. What are the nurse's responsibilities in relation to this problem?

9. Analgesic drugs may frequently be combined with each other or with drugs such as barbiturates. Why might this be a special hazard?

10. What nursing responsibilities may be utilized in avoiding the need for administration of sedatives and hypnotics?

11. What are some of the undesirable effects of sedatives and hypnotics, for which the nurse should be alert?

12. What are the indications for use of central nervous system stimulants? Give examples.

13. Distinguish between mydriatic and miotic.

14. Why are some mydriatics contraindicated in the presence of glaucoma, or in patients predisposed to glaucoma?

15. What are the major anatomic divisions of the autonomic nervous system?

16. What are some of the functions of the autonomic nervous system?

17. How are the divisions interrelated in funtions?

18. Epinephrine is an adrenergic drug. What are some of its actions? How is this drug administered?

19. What are the major uses of adrenergic drugs?

20. What are the major uses of adrenolytic drugs?

21. Acetylcholine mimics the effect of stimulation of the parasympathetic nervous system. What are some of these effects? What is the antidote?

22. What drug is best known for its parasympatholytic action? What are its uses? In what instances may this drug be contraindicated?

23. Give examples of drugs which may be included in the same group.

11

TREATMENT OF FEVER

The human body, as is the body of all the warm-blooded animals, is kept at a relatively constant temperature regardless of outside temperature. This is not the case with cold-blooded animals (fish, reptiles, insects, etc.) whose temperature ranges widely and corresponds closely with that of the outside environment. The human body temperature is kept warm at about 37 C. (99 F.) by complex mechanisms which are under the control of the brain. Briefly, constant temperature is maintained by a balance between heat formation and heat dissipation.

Body Heat

Heat is formed in the body by the burning (or utilization) of food and various other metabolic processes. These mechanisms for heat production do not respond readily to drugs, and when drugs act directly to depress the rate of heat formation it is usually a toxic reaction. On the other hand, mechanisms for heat formation in the body are highly sensitive to infectious processes (as well as some noninfectious processes) and body temperature rises in most infections.

The body constantly loses or dissipates heat. The rate at which it is lost is controlled by two devices; (1) by radiation of heat from the surface of the body much in the same way as any hot object cools off by radiating heat into the surrounding air, and (2) by the evaporation of perspiration much as the evaporation of water from the surface of a canteen bottle cools its contents. The rate at which heat is lost through radiation corresponds to the circulation of blood under the skin; the greater the cutaneous circulation, the

126

larger the amount of heat lost; conversely, decreased cutaneous circulation conserves body heat. The amount of heat lost by evaporation corresponds to the amount of sweat evaporated; this may be increased or decreased by alterations in the rate of perspiration. Usually the amount of heat lost by radiation exceeds that lost by evaporation.

In hot weather, or after strenuous exercise in which a great deal of heat is generated, the skin may become pink through increased cutaneous circulation and the amount of heat may increase to the extent that the person is literally drenched. In this way the internal temperature of the body may be kept cooler than that outside. In extreme cold when loss by radiation is rapid the body tries to conserve its heat and the reverse takes place: sweating ceases and the skin blanches because the cutaneous circulation is decreased.

Fever

When the temperature rises above normal in illness the question of treating the temperature as a symptom arises. This question is almost always pressed by the patient or his relatives because it is well known by the layman that high temperatures can be brought down by medication. Such medications are among the oldest, and the list of drugs which can do this is large. The tendency to reduce fevers in all cases was well established as a tradition in the era of medical practice when few drugs were known which could affect the cause of the disease. Since many physicians felt they should do something, indiscriminate reduction of fever became a common practice. Thus, it is often expected or even demanded of the physician that he do something about high temperature, despite the serious question of whether temperature reduction is a wise course in all illnesses.

There are some who now contend that fever is one of the body's defense mechanisms. Although there is little proof that this is the case, neither is there clear proof that fever, in itself, is harmful. In most cases fever is merely a symptom; at most it may cause some discomfort. Finally, there is evidence that heroic measures to reduce high fever abruptly may bring about vasomotor collapse.

The more modern attitude is to weigh the effect of the fever in the particular patient. Many physicians feel that the temperature curve is a useful guide to the course of an illness, and it should not be given up unless substantial gains are made in some way by reducing the fever with drugs. They point out that masking the fever curve with drugs may give everyone concerned a false sense of security. In instances in which the patient becomes restless or cannot sleep because of his fever, or when the fever is so high as to be dangerous, fever reduction seems indicated. In such cases there are physical and medical devices which may used.

The simplest devices are the physical ones. The patient can be sponged with cool water or alcohol, in which case he loses a considerable amount of heat by evaporation and radiation. In instances of very high temperatures, such as heat stroke, the patient may even be immersed bodily in a cold bath. Here the heat is lost by radiation (or conduction.) Such physical cooling devices leave the patient much more comfortable than do drugs, for the patient is clean while after drug administration he may be moist and sweaty.

There are no drugs which may be used safely to reduce the rate of heat formation, but there are a large number which safely increase the rate of heat loss. In general all the so-called simple analgesic drugs belong to this group of antipyretic drugs. The best known are the salicylates. It is interesting that while the usual therapeutic doses of these drugs have no influence on normal body temperature, their use in a fever is very effective. They produce this result both by increasing the rate of cutaneous circulation, thus increasing heat loss through radiation, and by increasing the rate of perspiration, thus increasing heat loss by evaporation. One result of the use of these drugs is excessive perspiration, a fact which requires nursing attention for the patient's comfort and health. Since they also relieve mild aches and pains and are relatively safe, they are frequently applied in simple and common infections by the layman without the advice of the physician.

In a sense, of course, the anti-infective drugs, when effective, reduce fevers by reducing heat formation, but this is not a direct action on the nervous mechanisms involved. It is, rather, a specific action on the cause of the infection. None of the so-called antipyretic drugs, such as the salicylates or acetophenetidin exert any effect on the course of the infection.

There are a few drugs which are used therapeutically to increase body temperature in the treatment of conditions which indicate that high temperature has a specific therapeutic value. Usually fever is induced by a reaction to foreign proteins. Such reactions produce startlingly high fevers with chills. Among the agents used for this purpose are typhoid vaccine, live malaria parasites and milk products. The hot box, a chamber in which the patient is enclosed with his head exposed, heats the patient externally and does not permit heat loss. In this manner it also raises the body temperature greatly.

Drugs Used in Treatment of Fever

Antipyretics	Pyretics
Diaphoretics	Sudorifics *see* Diaphoretics

Study Questions

1. How is body temperature maintained at a normal level?

2. In what ways may temperature elevation be of value?

3. How do antipyretic drugs reduce abnormally elevated temperatures?

4. How do the antipyretic drugs effect normal body temperature?

12

TREATMENT OF THE ALLERGIC STATE

Allergy is a state of specific hypersensitiveness which may exist in an organ or tissue of the body, most commonly the respiratory tract, the skin and the digestive system. In the allergic state, violent and extremely serious symptoms may develop as the result of exposure to minute amounts of substances which are entirely innocuous to normal persons even in large amounts. The exact manner in which hypersensitivities develop is highly technical and still a matter of dispute. It may, however, be stated simply that as a result of previous exposure to a substance which may be termed an "allergen" a "reagin" is produced in certain tissues which then become hypersensitive. The reagin is a reactive material which continues to be present in the tissues after exposure. On subsequent exposure to the allergen, the combination of the allergen with the reagin leads to the production of histamine or histamine-like substances which, in turn, produce the allergic symptoms in the tissue or organs in which this reaction takes place.

The allergens and reagins are highly specific, and in most instances neither will combine even with closely related allergens or reagins. In general, the most potent allergens are proteins which vary greatly in allergenic potency. Virtually any substance, however, may act as an allergen to induce allergic hypersensitivity. Thus, there are allergies to foods, pollens, drugs, clothing materials, dyes, chemicals, paints, upholstery materials, animal danders, plants, oils, etc.

It is unknown why certain people develop allergies upon exposure to a particular allergen, and why others, upon similar exposure to the same allergen do not. But it is clear that a familial

130

tendency to allergic disease exists. There also is substantial evidence that the allergic state in some patients may be heightened by emotional and stressful situations. There is also the interesting fact that although allergies tend to be highly specific, once an allergic reaction has been aroused, the hypersensitive states may temporarily extend to related allergens.

The allergic manifestations, and hence the disease, depend on the tissues in which the allergic reaction develops (or in which the specific reagin is present). Most common are: hay fever, allergy of the nasal mucous membranes; asthma, allergy of the muscle, glands and mucous membranes of the bronchi; urticaria, allergy of the blood vessels of the skin; angioneurotic edema, allergy of the blood vessels of the subcutaneous tissues; eczema, allergy of the epidermis of the skin. There are also allergies of the digestive mucous membranes, other forms of skin allergies, and probably many other allergic manifestations which are rarely identified.

The symptoms depend largely on the organ or tissue involved. Thus, there may be sneezing, tearing, swelling, coughing, wheezing, dyspnea, itching, eruptions, nausea, vomiting, cramps, etc. Treatment includes (1) identification of the specific allergen, (2) avoidance of the allergens, (3) desensitization, (4) antihistaminic drugs, (5) sympathomimetic drugs, (6) spasmolytic drugs, (7) ACTH and cortisone.

The identification of the allergen is not always a simple matter. In some instances the time, season and place may provide a clue. In some cases the allergen may be identified by elimination diets, changes in clothing, toothpastes, soaps, cosmetics, furniture stuffings, household pets and so forth.

Skin tests are often useful, especially in the case of contact and inhalation allergens. Too often, however, it happens that none of these means of exploration is useful, and specific treatment cannot be carried out. But when specific identification of the allergen is made, treatment may proceed along the lines of avoidance of the allergen. Often this is not practical or possible and other measures must be taken.

Allergenic Preparations

Allergenic preparations are extracts of substances for which a hypersensitivity may be present. These extracts may be made from countless different materials: pollens, hair, epidermis of animals, feathers, food, animal and vegetable fibers, plants, fungi, bacteria. These extracts are used for both diagnosis and treatment. In using them for diagnosis, sensitivity is determined by introducing a small amount of the allergen into the epidermis by a scratch or by intradermal injection. The development of a wheal, greater in size than that produced by a similar amount of the diluent alone (without the extract), is taken as a positive reaction and suggestive of the specific hypersensitivity. False positive and false negative reactions are relatively common.

Treatment of allergies is carried out by desensitization with the allergenic extracts. This process consists of a long series of injections, the first being so small as to cause no reaction, and each successive one increasing by an increment also too small to cause reaction, but serving to build up resistance. As sensitivity is depressed by this gradual process and the successive doses are increased, a practical degree of desensitization to the particular allergen may be developed. This process is helpful in about 75 per cent of all cases of inhalation allergy in which the allergen can be identified; it is much less successful in other allergic diseases. Desensitization never provides a permanent cure since the patient returns to his former state of hypersensitivity soon after the treatment lapses. In the case of seasonal allergies, however, desensitization may be repeated from year to year. The treatment, consisting as it does of many injections, is long, drawn out, disagreeable and expensive. It is also productive of unpleasant reactions. For these reasons the relatively new antihistaminic drugs, which provide many patients with relief by the oral administration of a tablet, are often tried before desensitization.

Antihistaminic Drugs

Antihistaminic drugs attack the product of the reagin-allergin reaction, histamine. When antihistaminics are given to an animal which has already reacted to histamine, the animal may be relieved of the most severe symptoms. Similarly, in a large proportion of patients these drugs may effectively relieve or prevent the symptoms of an allergic reaction. The mode of action of the antihistaminic drugs is strictly conjectural, but it may represent a competition between the histamine and the antihistamine drugs for the cells of the body.

Clinical reports of the action of antihistaminic drugs have been favorable in many of the varied allergic manifestations, urticaria, dermographism, atopic dermatitides, cold allergy, and pruritic states, hay fever (seasonal and nonseasonal) asthma, ocular allergies, gastro-intestinal allergies, Meniére's syndrome, serum sickness, drug reactions and in some instances of migraine headaches. There is no adequate explanation why the antihistaminic drugs are not effective in all allergic manifestations. Nevertheless, they are effective in a sufficiently large number of cases to warrant trial. The antihistaminic drugs, in particular dramamine, are being used with some success in the prevention and treatment of seasickness and dizziness in general.

The dangers of the antihistaminic drugs are few; there are some idiosyncrasies and even drug allergies to these antiallergic drugs. Many antihistaminics, like diphenhydramine (benadryl), induce drowsiness and exert an action so similar to that of the barbiturates that this must be guarded against in patients who pursue a skilled or dangerous occupation and even those who drive a car. There are occasional gastro-intestinal disturbances, but there have been few serious reactions.

A word should be said about the use of these drugs in the treatment of the common cold, a procedure very popular when these drugs were first introduced. The antihistaminic drugs exert no specific action against the common cold or its cause. There are, however, some patients in whom some symptoms may be due to an allergic reaction which develops during the cold and which prevails only during its active stages. The exact nature of the allergen in such a case is not known, but in such cases there is always the possibility that antihistaminic drugs may relieve the allergic aspects of the cold; how much relief depends entirely on how much of the entire picture of distress is due to the allergic aspects of the cold. Thus, the antihistaminic drugs will not provide any relief to some patients with colds, only a little to others, and a great deal to a few patients. They should not, therefore, be used indiscriminately in all cases, nor should good results be expected in many patients.

Sympathomimetic Drugs

Sympathomimetic drugs, epinephrine (adrenalin), ephedrine and the group of related drugs are potent antiallergic drugs. On the other hand, the antagonistic drugs, the vagomimetic drugs like methacholine and physostigmine, may precipitate attacks in patients with allergies, and as a matter of precaution they should be avoided whenever possible in such patients. The nature of these reactions, both the protective action of epinephrine and the precipitating action of methacholine is not clear, but the effects are often very dramatic. Thus a patient whose life is seriously threatened by an allergic attack may have his life saved by an injection of epinephrine, and a patient without symptoms may have a violent asthmatic attack as the consequence of a dose of methacholine given for some other condition.

Epinephrine is the most effective of all sympathomimetic drugs in this respect. It provides relief for urticaria, asthma, angioneurotic edema, serum sickness, anaphylactic shock and even hayfever. The importance of epinephrine in therapy has been somewhat reduced by the introduction of the antihistaminic drugs which are simpler and less disagreeable to use, but in the event of a grave emergency, epinephrine is still the drug of choice.

Along with its related drugs it has an important position, not only for the emergency in which there is no time to wait and no margin of safety for trial with a drug which may not work, but also for the relief it provides in cases in which the antihistaminic drugs have failed.

Epinephrine may be given by injection of the aqueous solution, the suspension of the oily product for long action, by direct application (drops or spray) to the nasal mucous membranes for decongestion, and by inhalation of the concentrated solution in the form of a nebulized (aerosol) spray. Overdosage may have serious ill effects and dosage should, therefore, be carefully measured. The solution used for nebulization is so strong (1%) that it must *never* be used for injection; it may prove fatal.

Epinephrine has disagreeable side actions; it elevates blood pressure, accelerates the heart, increases the work of the heart, causes anxiety and nervousness. Overdosages may be dangerous, especially in patients with hypertension or coronary artery disease. The related drugs, ephedrine and others, have the advantage of oral administration, and although they are not as rapid in action or as potent as epinephrine, they have a more persistent action and are not as disagreeable for the patient. These are more commonly used than epinephrine in cases which are not urgently in need of relief.

Recently, a derivative of epinephrine, isopropyl arterenol, has been introduced. This drug possesses the antiallergic and cardiac stimulant actions of epinephrine, but not its vasoconstrictor action. For this reason isopropyl arterenol may be used for the relief of allergic reactions without much of the disagreeable effects of epinephrine on the blood pressure.

Antispasmodics

Antispasmodics such as aminophyllin may be used in the treatment of acute asthmatic attacks. These drugs may relax the bronchial musculature which is in spasm in the asthmatic attack. For quick relief the aminophyllin may be given intravenously. It is well to remember in this emergency that when the drug is given by that route, it must be given slowly if serious reaction is to be avoided. Take especial note of the fact that the intramuscular preparation which is usually quite concentrated and contains some local anesthetic may cause serious reaction if given intravenously. For intravenous injection only the proper preparation, a pure and well diluted one, may be used.

In this condition epinephrine is also effective and may be useful in cases in which aminophyllin fails. It is to be recalled that epinephrine relaxes the smooth muscle of the bronchi.

Cortisone and Corticotropin (ACTH)

Cortisone and corticotropin (ACTH) may be used in allergic emergencies or may serve as adjuncts to other drugs in the treatment of serious or resistant allergic manifestations. At the present time, these drugs are not to be used routinely; they are indicated only in cases which have not responded well to the usual treatments, and in urgent situations such as status asthmaticus. These drugs have been found to be effective in resistant cases of allergic conjunctiv-

itis, herpes zoster opthalmicus, angioneurotic edema, atopic dermatitis, exfoliative dermatitis and drug reactions. Problems attending
their use are discussed elsewhere (page 212). Hydrocortisone is
effective by local application, and ointments containing this material may be applied successfully for allergic skin manifestations.

Drugs Used in Treatment of Allergy

Adrenergics	Antispasmodics
Antihistaminics	Decongestants (nasal)
Allergenic extracts	Hormones

Study Questions

1. By what process, in brief, is it believed that an allergic state may
be developed?

2. Indicate some of the major manifestations of an allergic reaction,
including symptoms.

3. What does the plan for treatment of allergies usually include?

4. In what ways are allergenic substances used?

5. What seems to be one of the significant untoward effects of many
of the antihistaminic drugs such as diphenhydramine?

6. Why may parasympathomimetic drugs be contraindicated in
patients known to have allergies?

7. Of what value are the sympathomimetic drugs in the treatment
of allergic states?

8. Aminophyllin is used in the treatment of acute asthmatic attacks. What is its action and what are special precautions to be taken
into consideration in its administration?

13_____

TREATMENT OF
NUTRITIONAL DISTURBANCES

The term nutrition has much broader implications than is generally appreciated. It implies not only the eating of foods, minerals, vitamins and the like, but also the food's conversion into materials which the body can use. Finally, nutrition implies the way in which the body uses the material it digests to maintain growth, replacement, activity and good health. This includes, therefore, not only digestive processes in the intestine, but also metabolic processes all over the body, chemical and physical processes which are involved in maintaining the various physiologic activities of the organs and tissues of the body, and its constancy, or to use the presently more fashionable term, homeostasis. Nutritional diseases may be divided into dietary, electrolyte and metabolic disturbances.

There are five major types of disturbances which can upset the body's homeostasis: (1) inadequate supply of the necessary nutritional elements, foodstuffs, vitamins, minerals, calories, etc.; (2) inadequate absorption of vital elements of nutrition; (3) abnormal losses by the body of elements of nutrition; (4) abnormal destruction in the body of nutritional elements; (5) abnormal metabolism or handling by the body of nutritional elements.

The symptoms in these disturbances can be widespread, involving either all or just a single organ of the body, and can produce a wide variety of symptoms depending on the organs involved. Among the symptoms one encounters are pain, malaise, fatigue, edema, weakness, neuritis, disturbances in cardiac rhythm, convulsions, collapse, defective bones, defective growth and defective healing of wounds. Treatment depends on the cause of the disturbance and the specific elements in the diet which may be deficient.

Inadequate Ingestion

The essential elements of the diet are (1) carbohydrate, (2) protein, (3) fat, (4) minerals, (4) vitamins and other accessory foodstuffs. Food must be adequate in the amount of calories it provides, as well as in the absolute amounts of essential elements. Inasmuch as in some cases the amount of one element ingested increases the need for the other (fat and carbohydrate, carbohydrate and vitamin B_1), the minimum amounts of each essential for health cannot be established without relating it to the amount of the others ingested. In any event, the materials ingested must be sufficient in amount and proper in relationships in order to supply the metabolic needs of the body and maintain homeostasis.

The results of inadequate ingestion are a kind of malnutrition which depends largely on the nature of the insufficiency. In chronic malnutrition due to poverty, the more expensive and commonly the more essential elements of the diet are inadequate in amount. These are protein, fat, vitamins and minerals. Under such conditions, while the patient may be overweight he is, nevertheless, undernourished; he eats large amounts of carbohydrate because it is cheaper, but he suffers from malnutrition due to insufficiency of the more vital elements of the diet. In rarer instances, the inadequacy is on a caloric basis while the essential elements such as proteins, minerals and vitamins are adequate in amount. When overweight people are on poorly controlled weight reduction schedules, there is a grave danger of the development of some type of insufficiency because of an improperly balanced diet.

A short statement should be made about the elements of food. Carbohydrate is the most abundant and cheapest food material we have. It is high in caloric value and, because it is concentrated and does not satisfy appetite as quickly as does fat or protein, people on a high carbohydrate diet tend to eat relatively large quantities of it. In small amounts, carbohydrate in the diet is essential for it assists in the complete utilization of fat. Beyond this required amount it merely supplies calories which, when present in excess, are converted to fat and stored as such in the body.

Protein is essential for maintaining the integrity of the organs and structures of the body, themselves being mainly composed of protein. In diets which lack sufficient protein materials the body drains its organs and muscles, consequently undermining the health of these structures. Fat is also essential in small amounts, but beyond this it supplies only calories. Since it is a relatively expensive food it is not as often the cause of obesity as carbohydrate food.

In the event of diets that are insufficient calorically the body first calls upon its fat stores for calories (there are no important carbohydrate stores). When these are consumed, the flesh of the body and the more vital organs are then utilized to supply the energy needs of the body.

In constructing a diet for the obese patient, caloric intake is cut down to a level below the energy requirements of the body but a sufficient amount of proteins, vitamins and minerals must be supplied for the body's metabolic needs. As a consequence, on such a properly adjusted diet, the organs and vital structures are protected, the body utilizes the fat depots for the energy requirements of the body and weight reduction occurs solely as the result of fat loss.

Vitamins and minerals are specific essential elements and there are no substitutes for them. It is for this reason that in constructing diets for patients for any reason whatever the body's needs for these essential elements must be fully satisfied.

It is difficult to place the symptoms of chronic alcoholism in relation to the type of nutritional disturbances found. In general, chronic alcoholism results in chronic malnutrition because the alcoholic tends to eat little when drinking, while at the same time the utilization of alcohol increases the body's need for vitamin B_1. It is for these reasons that vitamin deficiencies and neuritis are common in alcoholics.

The patient with hyperthyroidism may also be mentioned here; his caloric requirements are increased so far above normal by his disease that if he ingests only what a normal man of his size needs, he still has an inadequate intake. As a consequence, the patient with hyperthyroidism tends to lose weight. Usually, however, there are no specific deficiency symptoms in this condition.

Nutritional deficiencies are especially common and often serious in the infant and child whose needs for rapid growth are both great and critical. There is a corresponding nutritional situation in the pregnant female, whose requirements are also unusually great in order to provide for the developing infant.

Finally, in both acute and chronic non-nutritional illness, nutritional requirements may rise while appetite is impaired or precarious and malnutrition results as a consequence.

These special situations form a special problem which cannot be considered here in detail; since they represent insufficient ingestion they can, in general, be satisfied by oral nutrition, with the needed foods, vitamins and minerals.

Parenteral Feeding

There are, however, illnesses in which it is not possible to solve nutritional problems by oral feeding. After intestinal surgery and in cases of coma, for example, parenteral feeding may be necessary in order to prevent malnutrition. Available now are preparations of minerals, vitamins, carbohydrates, proteins and electrolytes which can be administered parenterally; this procedure is a commonplace in modern hospital practice. It is to be remembered that complete nutrition by this means has its practical difficulties and disadvantages. Complete nutrition by the parenteral route is almost impossible to achieve for a prolonged period of time. In practice the attempt is made to supply merely a part of the essential needs of the body by this route. Adequate caloric nutrition by the parenteral route requires exceedingly large amounts of fluid and the problem is an especially difficult one with protein. While there are now amino acid mixtures which provide the elemental form of protein and may be administered intravenously, there is also ample evidence that it is exceedingly difficult to maintain protein balance by this mode of feeding alone. There are, at present, no satisfactory means of supplying fat parenterally.

The simplest food to administer by any parenteral route is sugar. Sugar is cheap, soluble, sterilized by heat without destruction. Sugar, in its common form sucrose, is not utilized by the body if it is administered parenterally, and other sugars must be used for this route of administration. Dextrose (glucose) is well tolerated by tissues and blood in concentrations up to 20 per cent. Higher concentration may prove irritant and very high concentrations may cause venous thrombosis. A new addition to the available sugars is fructose or levulose. There is the suggestion that fructose is more readily available to the body than dextrose.

Inadequate Utilization of Food

In a number of diseases and illnesses food may be ingested in adequate amount and in proper balance but may not be normally utilized. A simple example is the patient who has frequent or persistent vomiting, for whom the food ingested provides nothing at all, and who in addition, soon suffers from the continued loss of electrolyte in the gastric juices expelled. A comparable situation exists with continued severe diarrhea in which food absorption may be incomplete because of the rapidity with which it moves along the intestine. This is also coupled with excessive losses of water and electrolyte (especially alkali).

In addition, there are specific deficiencies and illnesses in which the intestine, because of defects in digestive juices, is unable to prepare food for absorption, and as a consequence, much that is ingested passes out of the intestine without utilization. This is seen in serious disease of the liver when there may be insufficient bile to prepare fat for digestion; to make matters worse, the liver may not be able to participate in the utilization of absorbed proteins. As a consequence serious protein deficiencies may result in liver disease. The diabetic is another example of the person who cannot adequately utilize food: he cannot use sugar although he absorbs it well.

There are other disturbances which may interfere with the utilization of calcium for the formation of bones (insufficient vitamin D), iron for the formation of blood cells and so forth. In such illnesses, the primary disease must be corrected if it is to be cured, but in some cases, the ingestion of larger than normal amounts of the needed element may result in some utilization with relief of symptoms. In other cases such a procedure may be harmful. In some cases the parenteral, rather than the generally preferred oral administration of vital food elements may be a way of overcoming a difficulty in absorption.

Unusual Nutritional Loss

Unusual losses of nutritional elements from the body occur in many conditions, with the loss being great enough to produce serious deficiencies and symptoms resulting from it. In cases of vomiting and persistent diarrhea, already mentioned, there may be serious loss of electrolyte as well as ingested foodstuffs. After surgery and trauma, fluid electrolyte, and in some cases even body proteins, may be lost in large amounts resulting in serious symptoms. In kidney disease there may be serious loss of protein due to the persistence of albumin in the urine. In hemorrhage there may be critical losses of fluid and the formed elements of blood. In excessive perspiration the loss of sodium chloride may be great enough to produce severe cramps and weakness. With frequent paracenteses (tappings) of fluid from the abdomen or the chest, enough protein may be removed to produce serious depression of blood protein levels. The diabetic loses large amounts of ingested carbohydrate and may be undernourished as a result. Certain medications taken for long periods of time (mercurial diuretics producing excessive loss of sodium chloride for instance) may cause electrolyte deficiency.

Nutritional disturbances due to loss should be recognized as a possibility and corrected before they develop into a serious matter. The correction may sometimes be accomplished by the ingestion of exceedingly large amounts of the material being lost, but in most instances the problem is not so simply solved, and best results are achieved by the correction of the defect which causes it.

The exact dose of the material needed in some of the more serious cases may be difficult to determine. Blood counts indicating the degree of loss of blood are sometimes helpful in cases of hemorrhage; in some conditions such as shock due to burns, etc., there are formulas by which dosage of blood, plasma or fluid may be determined. In serious and acute deficiencies due to nutritional losses the parenteral route of administration may be the preferred one.

In the case of replacement, the attempt is made to replace the specific deficient material, protein, carbohydrate, vitamin, mineral or electrolyte, as the case might be.

Destruction of Nutritional Elements

Increased destruction of nutritional elements may occur as a result of acute or chronic disease of any type, infectious, degenerative or neoplastic, and in some metabolic diseases. Depending on the nature of the illness either specific deficiencies or general malnutrition may result. The latter is often seen after prolonged infectious disease or in cancer, whereas specific deficiencies such as anemia may be due to increased destruction of blood. Again, in many instances such deficiencies cannot be easily compensated simply by the oral administration of large amounts of food; the basic disease continues to prevent adequate nutrition. Once the illness is cured, however, the patient responds well to oral feeding and regains his former state of nutrition.

The nutrition of patients who are chronically ill and subject to malnutrition by the combination of poor appetite, poor utilization of food and increased destruction is a serious nursing problem. Often these patients must be urged to eat at every meal, their food must be well chosen and well prepared and their tastes must be pampered. In general, a high protein diet rich in minerals and vitamins is selected. But even with all these measures, the patients remain malnourished.

Intravenous feeding sometimes helps in nutrition but such a form of feeding is impractical for the patient who is ill for a long period of time. In some cases it is difficult to find a vein for intravenous feeding; in others one wants to have the few remaining veins for emergencies which may arise. In such a situation the use of hyaluronidase to facilitate the absorption from the subcutaneous tissues is a measure which should be borne in mind.

Electrolyte and Fluid Disturbances

The electrolyte consists of the various salts (sodium, potassium, calcium, chlorides, etc.) which are dissolved in the blood plasma and are necessary for homeostasis. Electrolyte and fluid disturbances deserve special consideration because they are exceedingly common in health as well as illness and because there may be serious consequences when they are overtreated.

In many diseases, disturbances develop in the fluid and automatically in the electrolyte balance of the body. Large amounts of fluids and one or more electrolytes are lost in excessive vomiting, diarrhea, after surgical operations, hemorrhage, excessive diuresis due to drugs, adrenal diseases, diabetes, poisonings, shock, burns, excessive perspiration, etc. The losses incurred in such disorders may be so great as to exceed the ability of the body to compensate and maintain homeostasis by drawing from its stores. Dehydration, acidosis and alkalosis are among the most common complications seen. In some conditions, large losses of sodium chloride occur. The loss of large amounts of protein may also cause serious symptoms, not only because of the protein loss as a food, but also because protein is important as a buffering material and in controlling osmotic relationships of body fluids. Death may ensue from these complications of disease unless they are corrected.

In making such readjustments, it is important to discover the precise nature of the disturbance in order to supply the needed materials, and to determine its extent in order to determine the proper dosage. In most instances these materials and fluids will be administered intravenously. In cases in which this route is impracticable, hyaluronidase may be used together with fluids given subcutaneously.

It is easily possible by overtreatment or by giving too much of only one of the needed elements, to cause a new situation urgently requiring still another kind of corrective treatment. The treatment of electrolyte and fluid disturbances requires considerable expertness in order to obtain the best result. In addition, these treatments are usually required in urgently ill patients in whom any error may be fatal.

Parenteral Fluids

Parenteral fluids are any fluids used for injection, but in the main the term is applied to solutions given in large amount for fluid, nutritional or electrolyte content.

Special mention must be made of the water used for parenteral administration. In addition to the necessity for bacteria-free water, so that no infections result from it, the water used for large parenteral injections must also be "pyrogen-free." Precisely what a pyrogen is, is not known, but it is a fact that ordinary sterile distilled water may cause febrile reactions. The fever is caused by pyrogen, the unknown substance. For this reason water used for parenteral fluids is distilled several times in special ways and filtered so that all pyrogens are removed. An intravenous injection or infusion, unless otherwise specified by the physician, should be given slowly to prevent nonspecific reactions which may result from the rate of introduction of any material into the bloodstream. In most instances it is possible to add dextrose to these parenteral fluids to provide nutrition.

Most standard parenteral solutions are based on the nature of so-called physiologic fluids, that is to say, they tend to resemble body fluid in concentration, osmotic tension, acidity (pH), electrolyte composition. Whereas ordinary physiologic saline contains only sodium chloride, such solutions as Ringer's and Hartmann's solutions more closely simulate body fluids and are therefore somewhat better tolerated. Solutions which are too dilute may destroy (hemolyse) red blood cells and cause serious reactions. For special reasons some parenteral fluids contain alkalinizing materials, such as sodium lactate or sodium citrate. In some special cases, such as low sodium syndrome, hypertonic (highly concentrated) saline solution may be used. In some cases hypertonic solutions of dextrose, or other sugar, as concentrated as 50 per cent are administered intravenously. These solutions are not used for nutritional purposes, but rather to reduce intracranial pressure. They must be administered with great care or severe venous thrombosis will ensue.

Overnutrition

Overnutrition is still another problem in nutrition. This is commonly thought of in terms of obesity alone. While obesity is a real problem, not only because of the physical appearance of the patient, but also because it is a risk to health, it is not the only problem in overnutrition. There are, of course, many instances in which simple overingestion or overeating produces acute digestive symptoms. There are a few cases in which specific overindulgence produces special symptoms. Plain tap water, taken in excessive amounts, may cause serious dehydration and prostration. This is a situation more common in infants than adults, but in the latter, such a result may be seen in the case of a steel mill worker who sweats a great deal and drinks large amounts of water. It is to prevent these effects that such workers are required to take salt tablets every time they drink water. The excessive use of sodium chloride in the patient with edema may produce serious symptoms of congestive failure, or may throw a well-compensated patient into heart failure. The excessive and unnecessary use of minerals and vitamins on rare occasions may lead to serious toxic effects.

Obesity, either glandular or psychologic, may be considered the result of an illness. The glandular cause is by far the less frequent, and can be treated specifically after the diagnosis is established. The simplest example of this is hypothyroidism. Unfortunately, although it is relatively easy to treat, it is rarely the cause of obesity. This answer to the obesity problem is often sought by fat people, who after basal metabolism tests have their hopes dashed for an easy solution of their problem with pills.

Most cases of obesity result from overeating. The tendency to overeat in the largest number of these patients cannot be solved unless the patient gets some sort of help in planning his meals, and solving his emotional needs for overeating.

The use of drugs such as amphetamine (benzedrine) to depress appetite, thyroid extract (for a patient with a normal thyroid gland) to increase the rate of weight loss, or any other drug device used for obese patients is dangerous unless carefully planned and followed by the physician.

Vitamins

Vitamins deserve special consideration because they are vital constituents of our diet and are so widely used. The need for vitamins has long been known. By definition a vitamin is an essential dietary element which is required only in minute amounts. It is the minuteness of the needs which distinguishes the vitamins from, let us say, the protein in our diet. Both are essential for health but the vitamins are needed only in tiny doses. There are a great many vitamins and the symptoms which a deficiency may produce depend on whether the deficiency is of one or of more than one vitamin. Some symptoms of vitamin deficiency are well established and certain diseases can be related to them: rickets, scurvy, beriberi, polyneuritis, pellagra, others and combinations of them.

Vitamin deficiency diseases and symptoms may be found as clearly identifiable conditions only in situations of extreme vitamin malnutrition. These are rarely seen, except in extreme poverty, unusual dietary circumstances, chronic disease, alcoholism and infants. In addition there are more diffuse and less specific symptoms which may possibly be due to relative insufficiency of these essential elements in our diet. The more diffuse and less precise symptoms may be more widespread and also more difficult to identify. While the real extent of such deficiencies cannot be determined it is certain that its importance has been greatly exaggerated by the manufacturers of vitamins.

For the vast majority of people now taking vitamins regularly, the vitamins are not needed or do no good. There are few instances in which vitamins are harmful, but in the majority of cases reporting improvement from nonspecific symptoms, the effect is almost certainly purely psychologic.

Nevertheless, there is an argument for taking of moderate doses of vitamins where clear indications do not exist. For one, there is no harm in the measure providing the cost does not deprive the patient of something else essential for his health, and providing he has

Table 3—Daily Requirements for Essential Vitamins

Vitamin	Daily Maintenance Dose	Standard Tablet or Capsule
Thiamin	2 mg.	10 mg.
Riboflavin	2 mg.	10 mg.
Niacinamide	20 mg.	100 mg.
Ascorbic Acid	50 mg.	300 mg.
Calcium Pantothenate	5 mg.	20 mg.
Pyridoxine	0.5 mg.	2 mg.
Folic Acid	0.25 mg.	1.5 mg.
Vitamin B_{12}	2 µg.*	4 µg.*
Vitamin A	5000 units	———
Vitamin D	400 units	———
Vitamin K	2 mg.	———

* Abbreviation for microgram (1/1000 of a milligram).

no delusion about the purpose of the vitamins. Secondly, such doses of vitamins provide a kind of insurance against the diffuse and undiagnosable vitamin deficiencies which may exist because of the unnatural nature of most of our diets, stored food, canned food, food ripened artificially, overcooked food, improper choice of foods and ingestion of alcohol. Providing these limitations are borne in mind the taking of polyvitamin capsules is not harmful—and they may occasionally be useful. Standards for the daily requirements of the essential vitamins have been set (table 3) and should serve as the basis of such prophylactic use.

Metabolic Disturbances

Diabetes Mellitus

Diabetes mellitus may be considered a nutritional, a metabolic and an endocrine disorder. It is a condition in which nutrition may be seriously impaired because the body is unable to utilize carbohydrate in the normal way, and as a consequence, it pours out of the body into the urine. In this respect diabetes is a metabolic and a nutritional disorder. The disease is due to the improper function of an endocrine gland, the Islets of Langerhans, which are buried in the pancreas, and which produces a hormone, insulin, which governs the utilization of carbohydrate. Thus it also is an endocrine disease.

Diabetes may be treated by diet and by the use of insulin. The insulin used in medicine is an extract of the pancreas of cattle and it performs the same function when injected as the insulin normally produced in the body. Since insulin is not absorbed from the stomach it must be injected to be effective. The arrangement of the diet and the dose of insulin are usually in the hands of the physician and dietician. The nurse may administer the insulin and usually has to explain to the patient how to inject himself.

The effects of insulin are not always good: poor results and toxic reactions occur when the dose is improperly measured, when it is excessive and when the patient fails to eat. When there is an overdosage the insulin acts in the absence of carbohydrate to burn up the normally present sugar in the bloodstream. As a result the blood sugar levels become low and cause symptoms of hypoglycemia or insulin shock. This is characterized by nervousness, progressing into overactivity, confusion and coma. It is easily relieved in the conscious patient with sugar or orange juice.

There are several forms of insulin available, differing mainly in their speed of action. The purpose of the slowly acting insulins is to make it possible for a patient to get along with one injection a day.

Arteriosclerosis

Arteriosclerosis and diet have long been discussed and investigated as related phenomena. From time to time special diets have been constructed in the vain hope that they would control the development of this disease. More recently, cholesterol has been accused of being the culprit in this matter and at the present time there is considerable debate about its importance. It is true that blood cholesterol rises in conditions associated with arteriosclerosis but it is not clear which is the cause and which the effect. This is an especially pointed argument since it is clear that the cholesterol in the diet is not the same cholesterol as that which is found in the blood, and that the body is capable of forming large quantities of cholesterol even when it is completely deprived of it in food. The matter that should be considered when thinking of a low-cholesterol diet is the fact that such a diet is unappetizing and few people would be willing to undergo the ordeal of having it as a permanent fixture in their life if they knew how uncertain its importance is at this time. There are no drugs for the prevention or treatment of arteriosclerosis. Drugs are used only in the relief of the effects of the arteriosclerotic process on the various organs of the body.

Liver Disease

The liver is the largest and most complex organ of nutrition. Everyone recognizes that bile is formed in the liver and excreted through the bile ducts into the intestine. Bile is essential in the digestion of fat. But in addition, the liver is concerned with the other vital functions of metabolism of protein and fat, hemoglobin, cholesterol, blood clotting. Liver disease, therefore, may produce widespread and serious symptoms. Acute and chronic liver disease is characterized by jaundice, anemia, digestive difficulties, weakness, fever, malnutrition. It may result from infections, alcoholism, degenerative processes, vitamin and nutritional deficiences, drug reactions and from completely mysterious causes. Treatment consists of administering supportive therapy and directly treating the cause when it can be found. The supportive therapy usually consists of a highly nutritious diet, often high in protein, although notions vary, high-vitamin content, and often with injections of liver extracts. More recently much attention has been given to so-called lipotropic agents whose metabolism seems to be seriously disturbed in chronic liver disease. As a result, methionine and choline are given in exceedingly large (far greater than normal) amounts. With such therapy a few patients with the most extensive type of liver damage may improve. In general, the outlook for patients with advanced liver disease is very poor.

Gout

Gout is a metabolic disturbance of a specific substance, uric acid. For some reason the body does not handle this material well in a case of gout and tends to deposit it in and around joints where it causes exquisite pain and eventually begins to destroy the bone at these sites. The uric acid deposits of gout apparently do not depend entirely on outside sources, such as food, for in cases in which the uric acid in the diet is severely limited, the gouty process may still continue unabated.

The treatment of this unusual disorder is unsatisfactory because, as already stated, measures for limiting uric acid intake may not be effective. We do have drugs such as cinchophen, which increase the rate of uric acid elimination, but they too are not very effective in controlling the disease. Within the past few months a new drug, probenecid (benemid), has been introduced. Although it is said to increase uric acid excretion and to relieve pain, claims for it are not yet fully substantiated. There is some success in the treatment of gout with cortisone and corticotropin (ACTH). Finally, there is the important fact that the cause and basic nature of gout is not understood. In most instances the effective measures in gout are those which are directed against the pain.

Drugs Used in Treatment of Nutritional Disorders

Electrolytes, *see* Parenteral fluids   Lipotropics
Food preparations   Parenteral fluids

Study Questions

1. What major types of disturbances may effect homeostasis?

2. What factors affect the nutritional needs of the individual?

3. Give examples to illustrate instances of inadequate utilization and loss of nutritional substances.

4. Indicate some conditions and circumstances which may result in electrolyte and fluid disturbances.

5. What are "pyrogen-free" solutions?

6. What special factors should be considered in the treatment of obesity?

7. Why is insulin administered parenterally?

8. What are the nurse's responsibilities in the administration of insulin and the instruction of patients with diabetes regarding insulin?

14

TREATMENT OF
CARDIOVASCULAR DISORDERS

Diseases of the cardiovascular system are the most common as well as the most important diseases of man. There has been a huge increase in the incidence of these diseases, largely the result of the fact that the span of life has been increased by public health measures. Many more people than ever before live long enough to develop arteriosclerosis and hypertension and the heart disease which so frequently follows. This situation in a way provides a new problem because these diseases tend to be chronic to a large extent. The patients undergo a long period of partial or complete disability, requiring a great deal of medical and nursing skill and attention. Because of its chronic character and high incidence, medical care is often placed largely in the hands of the nurse with less than average supervision by the physician. Thus the role of the nurse and her understanding of the treatment of this illness—the biggest and broadest problem in medicine today—has become more important than ever.

The heart is not only a crucial organ, disease of which may threaten the life of the patient, but its efficiency is vital to the function of every organ and in heart disease symptoms may develop in any organ of the body. As a consequence treatment is complex and the list of drugs used is long. It is for this reason that a proportionately larger section of this book is devoted to the treatment of these diseases.

The cardiovascular system consists of the heart which pumps blood, and a system of blood vessels (arteries, capillaries and veins) which conduct blood to and from the various organs, bringing it into intimate contact with the cells that comprise the organs and

152

tissues. Drugs used in the treatment of this complex system may be divided into three categories: (1) those which act primarily on the heart, (2) those which act primarily on the blood vessels and (3) a large group of miscellaneous drugs used for the relief of related symptoms in heart disease but which have no important direct actions on either the heart or the blood vessels. This last group will receive brief mention here and more detailed consideration in appropriate sections.

Heart disease in the young is either congenital (that the patient is born with) or due to rheumatic fever. In older people it is more often caused by arteriosclerosis, hypertension, syphilis, or hyperthyroidism. Other types of heart disease are uncommon.

Drug Actions on the Heart

A brief description of heart action as well as the nature of some of its disturbances may be useful for an understanding of how drugs can exert a beneficial influence. The amount of blood pumped by the heart is determined by (1) the rate and rhythm of the heartbeat, and (2) the amount of blood expelled with each contraction of the heart. The rate of the heartbeat is normally controlled by a nervous or reflex mechanism, which accelerates or decelerates the heart rate in response to the demands of the body for blood. This mechanism regulates the rate of stimulus formation in the right auricle where impulses for the heartbeat are normally initiated. The rhythmically produced impulses pass down the auricles, and then to the ventricles through a specialized conducting system in the heart muscle (called the "bundle of His") which functions much as a nerve. In response to these impulses, first both auricles, and then both ventricles, which form the more important part of the pumping system, contract.

The normal conduction of these impulses results in an efficient coordination of the contractions of both auricles and both ventricles. In abnormal states the heart rate may be too rapid or it may be too slow, the regular rhythm may be replaced by partial or total irregularity, or there may be no coordination between the auricles and ventricles. Digitalis, quinidine, procaine, epinephrine (adrenalin) and other sympathomimetic drugs, methacholine and other parasympathomimetic drugs have been used to treat disturbances in rate and rhythm of the heart.

Insufficient output of the heart may be the result of decreased force of contraction of the heart, deficient filling of the heart, or a defect in the valves of the heart. Decreased force of contraction is usually the result of disease. Deficient filling is often due to mechanical interference. The third type of defect, that of the valves, is most often due to infectious disease. In this case the forward passage of blood may be incomplete because the valves cannot open completely or because, after contraction of the heart, blood flows backward past valves that cannot close completely. The digitalis glycosides are the only drugs that, in therapeutic doses, may be used to increase the force of contraction of the heart. There are no drugs that can repair damaged valves or increase deficient filling due to mechanical interference.

When heart muscle deteriorates as the result of disease or other defects that seriously impair cardiac function, congestive failure may result. In this state, the amount of fluid that lies between the cells and the capillary bed increases, sometimes to the extent of causing perceptible swelling (edema). This may develop in any or all organs, but is usually first noted in the ankles. Often it occurs in the liver, the abdominal cavity (ascites), the lung (pulmonary edema) or the pleural cavity (pleural effusion). Not all the factors that contribute to the development of this state are known, but the importance of some of them is clear. The pumping action of the heart may not remove blood rapidly enough from the great veins, thus causing a discrepancy between the rate of flow of blood from the heart and the rate of return from the body to the heart. As a result of this, blood accumulates in the veins, there is increased pressure in the capillaries, and more than normal amounts of fluid filters from the capillaries into the space between them and the cells. In addition, heart disease may adversely affect kidney circulation and prevent the kidneys from eliminating sodium in the urine. In the case of the seriously damaged heart the elimination of sodium in the urine may be reduced to a gram or even less per day, whereas with an average diet the patient may ingest from 10 to 15 Gm. of sodium. The retained sodium, holding water to maintain osmotic equilibrium with the fluid in the cells, is thought to be an important factor in the development of edema. In addition to edema, the symptoms of the weakened heart may include severe dyspnea, cyanosis, fatigability.

Drug Actions on Blood Vessels

The arteries, capillaries and veins form the bed for the blood that flows through the body. This bed has a far greater capacity than the total amount of blood in the body. Vascular dynamics are maintained at normal levels not only by the rate at which blood is pumped into the bed by the heart but also by a mechanism that keeps the vascular bed partially closed at all times. Some of the vessels are kept almost entirely closed, and in the others, tone is high so that the caliber of the vessels is relatively small. By this means the functional capacity of the vascular bed is kept equivalent to the amount of blood in it. By a change in these relations, large amounts of blood may be shifted from one area to another, from one organ to another, to meet special demands of the body. For example, during digestion, blood to the intestinal tract flows there in larger than usual amounts to supply the requirements of the digestive process, the vascular bed there being kept relatively open for this purpose.

If the tone of blood vessels throughout the body is great, there is marked resistance to the flow of blood and the heart is forced to pump against an excessively high blood pressure. If, on the other hand, as in the case of secondary or surgical shock, a relatively large part of the vascular bed opens at one time, the head of blood pressure falls precipitously, and vital mechanisms that depend on normal circulatory dynamics are threatened. In some diseases specific blood vessels may exhibit abnormally increased tone, to the extent that the blood flow to the part of the body affected is markedly impaired. This is the case in angina pectoris, in which a spasm of a coronary artery reduces the blood supply to a portion of the heart muscle and produces serious as well as painful symptoms. A blood vessel may be obstructed by a blood clot, and in such a case the condition may be further aggravated by vascular spasm, which the clot itself induces.

Drugs are used to increase or decrease the tone of blood vessels, to contract or dilate them. The constrictors are epinephrine and other sympathomimetic drugs, and the extract of the posterior lobe of the pituitary gland. The dilators are the sympatholytic drugs, the nitrites, papaverine and some tissue extracts. In addition, in the state of secondary shock, in which there is widespread dilation of the capillary bed together with a compensatory contraction of the arterioles, the condition is best alleviated by the addition of fluid to the total volume of blood for the functionally enlarged vascular bed. For this purpose, whole human blood, blood plasma, blood serum or a blood substitute such as an expander may be used.

Drug Action on Cardiac Symptoms

The symptoms of heart disease are pain, respiratory distress in a variety of forms, edema, fatigue, and disturbances in cardiac rhythm.

Cardiac Pain

Cardiac pain, one of the severest experienced in any disease, may come on suddenly in an attack and be exceedingly resistant to treatment. It may be the result of a sudden cardiac infarction, a spasm of a blood vessel, an inflammation of the pericardium, or a functional disturbance in which the coronary arteries fill poorly.

Cardiac pain is often associated with great anxiety on the part of the patient as well as those around him. The patient's restlessness and distress may appear to be aggravating his cardiac condition and, as a result, the measures used to relieve the pain often are heroic. It is for this reason that accidents due to overdosage with morphine occur while relieving the severe and resistant pain of an acute coronary infarction. It is well to bear in mind that morphine is, among other things, a potent respiratory depressant, and that in a patient with heart disease interference with respiration may have especially serious consequences. The dangers of serious overdosage should always be borne in mind when repeating doses of narcotic drugs in cases of severe and resistant cardiac pain. In many of these cases it is advisable to be satisfied with easing the patient's anxiety with the opiate rather than trying for nothing less than complete removal of the pain. In instances of less severe pain, complete relief can be obtained with safe doses of morphine or methadon, and sometimes meperidine (demerol) or codeine.

Anginal Pain

Anginal pain due to spasm of the coronary arteries may often be simply relieved with the use of the nitrite drugs. These drugs may also be used to prevent attacks of pain in circumstances of strain and stress which previous experience with the patient indicates are certain to induce an attack of angina.

Nitrites

The most commonly used of the nitrites are nitroglycerin, amyl nitrite and erythrityl tetranitrate. All have the same action, the only differences being in the speed and duration of the action. These materials, when taken by normal individuals, cause a sharp depression of blood pressure with faintness, giddiness, and severe headache, but in a case of angina pectoris, the proper dose relieves the pain without any side effect.

Usually the duration of the action is brief, although prolonged effects have been claimed. To the sufferer, the most desirable quality is the speed of relief. Amyl nitrite is about the speediest. It comes in small pearls which when broken just before using permit the vapors to be inhaled. It is best to break the pearl in a piece of gauze or handkerchief which is then held over the nose. Since the odor is particularly unpleasant and noticeable, it proves to be a great nuisance. The procedure is conspicuous and is impractical for the patient who daily requires a large number of doses which he must use in public.

The nitroglycerin comes in tiny tablets which are placed under the tongue and permitted to dissolve there; they are not swallowed. The effect comes on in a minute or less, almost as promptly as with amyl nitrite. The tablet can be taken without trouble (no water is necessary for swallowing) and without attracting any attention should they be required in a public place.

The nitroglycerin is taken in doses of from 0.2 to 0.6 mg. (gr. 1/300 to gr. 1/100). Although compressed tablets are often dispensed, the effects of the hypodermic tablets, taken under the tongue, come on more rapidly because they break up more readily. Since rapidity of action is desired, the hypodermic tablet should always be used. Patients usually carry small bottles of these tablets with them wherever they go, and some may take as many as 20 or more during a day. Nitroglycerin tablets deteriorate and lose potency with time.

Another material used for the treatment and prevention of the pain of angina pectoris is khellin (visammin). After trial in this country, conflicting reports on its usefulness have appeared. Some investigators claim that it is not much more effective than a placebo; others ascribe real relief to it. It must be remembered that there is a large psychologic element in the relief of the pain of angina pectoris, and that virtually anything, including a placebo, may give some degree of relief for a time. No drugs are as dependable or as effective as the nitrites for the treatment of the pain of angina pectoris.

From time to time other drugs will undoubtedly be introduced for the relief of anginal pain. At the time of this writing there are no drugs which are more dependable for the average patient with angina than the nitrite drugs, and any new remedy must be measured against them before it is accepted as an effective and useful drug.

Congestive Heart Failure

This condition is also commonly called heart failure and congestive failure. Most of the symptoms of heart disease other than the acute pain of coronary artery and inflammatory disease and cardiac arrhythmias may be considered to be due to cardiac insufficiency. In the sense that the symptoms are due to the fact that the heart fails to meet the demands which the body places on it, these symptoms may be said to be due to heart failure, and since congestion is a result, congestive heart failure. Most commonly, heart failure is considered in terms of intensely swollen ankles and great difficulty in breathing. These are the advanced stages of congestive heart failure, but there are also much earlier stages and milder symptoms. The list of symptoms is long and disagreeable: dyspnea, cyanosis, orthopnea, pain, palpitations, cough, edema, weakness, fatigue, pulmonary edema, etc. The commonest forms of treatment include (1) rest to reduce the burden on the heart, (2) reduction of salt (sodium) intake to reduce the tendency to accumulate fluid in the tissues (edema), (3) digitalis to increase the force of contraction of the heart and (4) diuretics to increase the excretion of fluid accumulated in the tissues.

Heart failure is a common and important syndrome, and the drugs used in it as well as the approach to treatment are widely discussed and argued. For these reasons the digitalis and diuretics which are usually the primary tools in treatment also hold the center of discussion; they are given especially thorough and detailed consideration here.

Digitalis and Digitalis Materials

Digitalis is the oldest and perhaps the most used of the effective drugs still in common use in the treatment of heart disease. Digitalis materials are very common in nature. They are present in a large number of plants. The entire group of drugs is called the digitalis group, and their purified extracts are known as the digitalis glycosides, regardless of the plant of their origin. The action on the heart is the same in the case of each digitalis drug. The differences between them are in (1) potency, (2) degree of absorption from the gastro-intestinal tract, (3) speed of action, (4) speed of elimination and (5) intensity of local irritant action in the gastro-intestinal tract. Although a number of different digitalis materials are considered in the pages which follow, only digitalis itself is discussed in detail. In the case of the individual drugs, only the differences between them and digitalis are discussed. The cardiac actions are listed as the properties of digitalis, but this applies to all the other members of the digitalis group.

Digitalis is obtained from the leaf of foxglove, or *Digitalis purpurea*, a plant commonly found in flower gardens. The strains used for the manufacture of the drug are selected to yield a large amount of digitalis glycoside, whereas the garden varieties are grown for the size and beauty of the flower. The leaf of the plant may be dried, ground, and pressed into tablets. *Digitalis tablets* is the form which is still most commonly used in medicine. An extract may be made with alcohol, *Digitalis tincture*, which is also a common form of medication. Some other extracts and some highly purified materials are listed later. The therapeutic actions are the same.

Actions: Digitalis exerts its principal actions directly on the

ACTION OF DIGITALIS

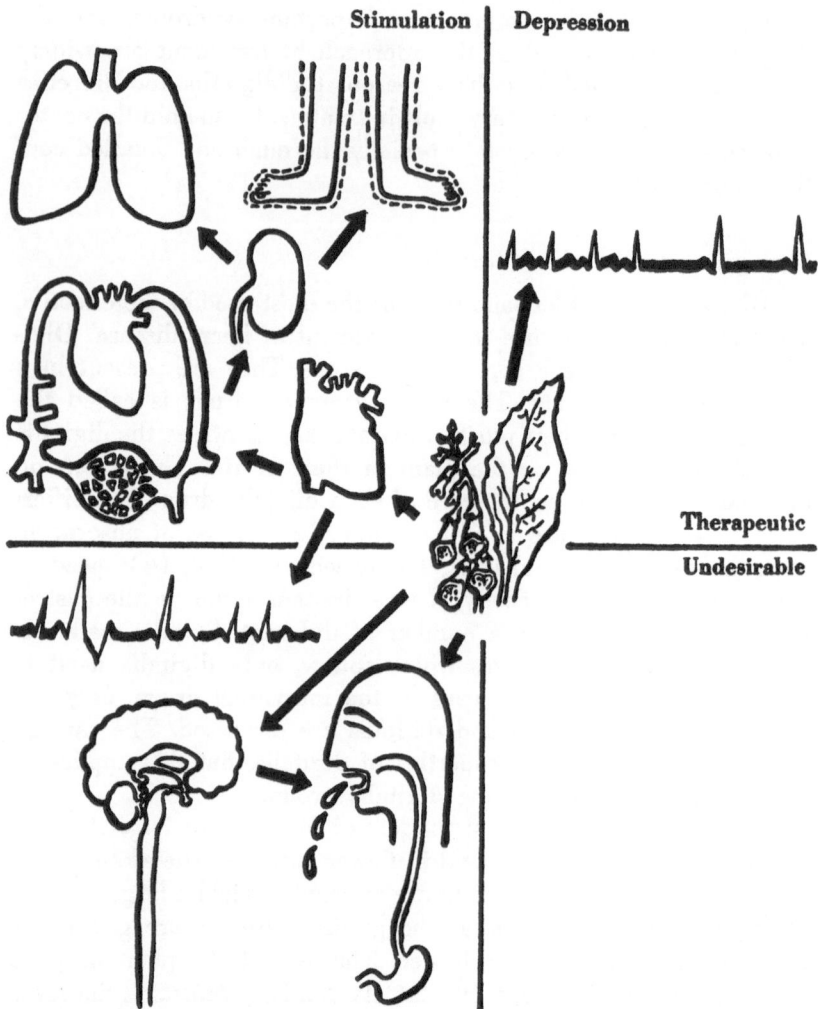

Fig. 8—All the therapeutic effects of digitalis derive from its cardiac actions: increase in force of contraction and slowing of heart rate. As a consequence of these, in patients with heart failure, urination may increase, edema disappear and respiration become more efficient. Toxic doses of digitalis may produce cardiac irregularities and induce vomiting by local and central actions.

heart. Some investigators claim important actions on the vascular bed of the liver as well. There are a large number of separate actions on the heart, but from the therapeutic standpoint the important effects are (1) increase in the force of contraction of the ventricle, and (2) depression of conduction through the bundle of His. In addition, digitalis has toxic actions of importance, chief of which are (1) local irritant action in the gastro-intestinal tract (nausea and vomiting are symptoms), (2) a systemic toxic action (which also produces nausea and vomiting) and (3) an action on heart muscle (whereby the muscle's rhythmicity is increased, thus producing disorders of rhythm).

Digitalis is the only drug (or group of drugs) in medicine which can increase the strength of the contraction of the heart; thus, it increases the ability of weakened heart muscle to pump blood. As a result of this effect, signs of congestive failure are relieved, the rate of urine production increases and a heart which is very rapid (in order to compensate for inefficiency) becomes slower.

Digitalis also exerts an action on the conduction of impulses from the auricle through the bundle of His to the ventricular muscle. This action is not often perceptible in the case of normal sinus rhythm, but it is a prominent action in the case of auricular fibrillation.

In auricular fibrillation, impulse formation in the auricle is rapid (often over 400 per minute), irregular and exceedingly variable in intensity. The ability of digitalis to depress conduction in the bundle of His (making it more difficult for impulses to pass through the bundle) screens the auricular impulses, rejecting the weak ones and permitting only the stronger ones to come down to the ventricle. As the digitalis action becomes more intense, the rate of the ventricle becomes slower (although, as may be seen in the electrocardiogram, the auricular rate is not slowed). The ventricular contractions become less variable in intensity and the rhythm more regular. Thus, an exceedingly rapid and inefficient ventricular rate of, say, 180 or 200, may be slowed to a normal rate of about 65 to 85. It is widely believed that this effect increases the efficiency of the heart (1) by permitting the slower ventricle to fill more efficiently with blood between contractions, (2) by relieving the ventricular muscle of the burden of the useless feeble contractions and (3) by permitting the slower ventricle more time for recovery between contractions. This effect of digitalis in auricular fibrillation is one of its most dependable ones, and it operates in addition to the effect of digitalis directly on the heart to increase the force of its contraction. Digitalis cannot, however, be counted on to slow the ventricular rate in all forms of tachycardia. In ventricular tachycardia the use of digitalis is dangerous.

Digitalis changes the electrocardiogram. This effect is of no practical value as an indication of the degree of digitalization of the patient. On the other hand, it is an action which often confuses diagnosis, for similar changes may occur in coronary thrombosis. The presence of digitalis effects in the electrocardiogram must be considered and accounted for, or important errors in diagnosis will be made. If digitalis is taken by the patient, a note to that effect should always be indicated on an order for an electrocardiogram.

Indications: There are two outstanding therapeutic indications for digitalis: heart failure and the rapid heart of auricular fibrillation. In the vast majority of these cases in which digitalis is indicated, the patient will require the drug for the remainder of his life.

Toxic effects: It is a matter of the first importance for nurses to understand and be aware of the nature of the undesirable effects of digitalis. The bad effects are frequently encountered, often overlooked and just as frequently thought to be present when the symptoms are due to another cause. It would be most unfortunate if a patient were deprived of this valuable drug because a mistake was made in the identification of a symptom. On the other hand, it would be equally unfortunate to harm a patient by the failure to recognize the earliest signs of digitalis intoxication. Properly used, digitalis is one of the safest of the effective drugs in the pharmacopeia. In under-dosage it is useless, in overdosage it may kill. A nurse's enlightened vigilance may make the difference.

The undesirable actions are usually divided into what are called minor toxic actions and major toxic actions. The minor toxic actions may be considered as warning signals which cause distress but no real harm. The minor toxic symptoms which the nurse may detect are (1) nausea and vomiting, (2) yellow spots or yellow discoloration of vision (xanthopsia), (3) premature contractions and (4) coupled rhythm (especially in the case of auricular fibrillation). In addition, a prolonged A.V. conduction can be seen in the E.C.G.

After the dose of digitalis is administered, a few minutes or many hours (as long as 12) may elapse before the nausea develops. In the case of an oral dose, nausea soon after the dose is likely to be due to an irritant action in the gastro-intestinal tract, whereas nausea which develops hours after the oral dose may be due to either local or systemic action. Nausea which develops after a parenteral dose of digitalis can only be due to its systemic action. It must be borne in mind that other causes, which may vary from a simple gastro-intestinal upset to an attack of coronary thrombosis, can produce nausea. It is important to know how to distinguish digitalis nausea in the patient who is receiving and needs the drug. If a patient does not lose his appetite but vomits or complains of nausea, the nurse may be quite certain that it is not digitalis nausea. Appetite is always impaired with digitalis nausea. If a patient has had the same daily dose of the same digitalis preparation for a month or more, nausea that appears is not likely to be digitalis nausea.

If a patient receiving digitalis complains of yellow vision, or if his pulse shows occasional irregularities, or in a case of auricular fibrillation, if the ventricular rhythm begins to couple or the rate becomes very slow (less than 60), digitalis intoxication may be suspected. The apical rate reveals such effects of digitalis and is always preferable to the pulse rate.

The advanced or major toxic symptoms are usually related to disorders of rhythm. If digitalis dosage is not adjusted, a few premature beats or coupled beats may gradually progress into a serious disorder of rhythm (ventricular tachycardia), or the slowing of the heart in auricular fibrillation may continue until a complete heart block with a ventricular rate of 30 is produced. Any alteration in rhythm during the course of digitalis therapy may be significant and should be brought to the doctor's attention at once.

There is no established antidote for digitalis poisoning but recent evidence seems to point to potassium. The more usual procedure is to stop the drug and wait and hope for sufficient elimination from the body before serious effects develop. As digitalis is slowly eliminated this waiting period may be a long and harrowing one for all concerned. Supportive therapy should be applied if it seems indicated, but the outstanding fact is that there is no specific remedy. In serious poisoning, the symptoms arise from the drug already absorbed. Washing the stomach is often of little use in such a case because the symptoms develop long after absorption in the gastro-intestinal tract is complete. The position of the nurse, therefore, is crucial in the detection of the signs of overdigitalization before serious intoxication develops through the uninterrupted use of digitalis.

Absorption and elimination: Digitalis is slowly and poorly absorbed from the gastro-intestinal tract. Only about 20 per cent of the glycosidal content of the whole leaf is absorbed. Digitalis is usually given orally, but in urgent cases the proper preparation may be given intramuscularly or intravenously. The drug is also absorbed from the rectum and may be given rectally to a patient who is vomiting.

Even after parenteral administration, digitalis develops its full effects slowly, perhaps 6 to 10 hours after the injection. The drug is also slowly eliminated from the body. After full digitalization, about two weeks are required for effects to be completely eliminated. Because of its slow elimination, only a single dose daily is required in a patient in whom it is desired to maintain digitalis action.

Potency: The potency of digitalis is expressed in terms of biologic units. Actual weight is not an accurate measure in this case, because the composition of the leaf varies from specimen to specimen, depending on the variety of the plant, the sunlight, rain, soil, and other conditions to which the growing plant was exposed and some unknown factors. As a result there are wide differences in the potency of specimens, and one specimen of digitalis leaf may be as much as two or three times as potent as another. There is no satisfactory chemical test and digitalis potency, therefore, is determined by bio-assay, or its effectiveness in a test animal. The animal may be a cat, pigeon, frog, or man. The potency of batches of digitalis on the heart is compared with that of a standard preparation in these test animals. The composition of the batches is altered until they equal in potency that of the U.S.P. standard material. An acceptable preparation contains the equivalent of 1 U.S.P. digitalis unit in 0.1 Gm., or 1 unit in 1.0 cc. of the tincture. Thus, there is a reasonable similarity in the potency of digitalis in all parts of the country.

Recently a method was devised for testing digitalis potency in man, using the effect of the electrocardiogram as an indication of cardiac action. This is an especially useful method because it takes into account absorption of the digitalis from the human gastrointestinal tract, and because the effectiveness of digitalis is tested in the species of animal which uses the drug therapeutically. The unit is designated as the *Human Unit* and is used by the New York Heart Association.

Dosage: The dosage regimen with digitalis depends on whether the patient has recently (within two weeks) had any digitalis. If he has not, the full digitalizing dose may be used. If digitalis has been used recently, the dose must be altered accordingly. Digitalis leaf is not usually given in one dose for digitalization because a large amount of irritant material is contained in the mixture and because the patient's tolerance or sensitivity to the local or systemic actions of digitalis has not yet been established. For these reasons, the full dose is usually divided into several parts (from 3 to 6) and given during the course of 12 to 24 hours, according to one of many schedules. Between doses, the patient is examined for untoward effects of the digitalis. If any are present, the scheduled dose is omitted. By such a program, toxic effects are avoided or minimized, while full digitalis action is obtained in 24 hours or less.

The total digitalizing dose varies with individual sensitivity and tolerance, from about 1.2 to 2.0 Gm. of the leaf, or from 12 to 20 cc. of the tincture. The maintenance dosage needs to be determined by trial. A dose is found which neither intensifies the effect nor permits it to diminish. This dose usually lies between 0.1 to 0.2 Gm. daily, or 1 to 2 cc. of the tincture. In terms of Human Units, the digitalizing dose is from 12 to 20 units, and the maintenance dose is from 1 to 2 units.

It is a matter of the first importance to determine the proper digitalis dosage. Once established, the maintenance schedule rarely needs changing, and no changes should be made by the nurse without instruction from the physician. The nurse should remember that digitalis action is so slow to develop that a delay of an hour or so will not influence the course of its action. If any question arises about the medication, there is, therefore, sufficient time for the nurse to get instructions from the doctor. Digitalis is not a drug to be given at odd times because of a whim, a hope or desperation.

Proper digitalization implies an adequate initial digitalization and an adequate maintenance regimen. Nothing haphazard will be either therapeutically useful or safe. Sudden changes in the patient's condition, such as a sudden attack of cardiac distress, are not likely to be helped in any way by a single additional dose of digitalis. In an urgent situation digitalis should not be used unless specific orders for its use have been left.

Digitalis is a safe drug when used properly. Tolerance and idiosyncrasy rarely develop. Changes in maintenance dosage are needed only when the condition of the heart changes. Digitalis may be taken for an unlimited number of years without danger of addiction or ill effect to any organ or physiologic system.

Other Digitalis Materials

Although all of the desirable therapeutic actions of digitalis may be satisfactorily obtained by the oral administration of the tablet of the crude leaf, and in the largest number of cases this is still the form used, there has been a growing tendency to use purified materials. The reasons for the change to purified materials are: (1) Pure materials are relatively constant in potency and may be administered in units of weight, whereas the cruder materials vary in potency, they must be assayed biologically (which at best is inaccurate), and dosage must be expressed in terms of biologic units. (2) Bio-assay usually provides no information on absorption and elimination. Potency and absorbability are constant in pure preparations, but are variable in the cruder materials. (3) The pure crystalline materials often have less local irritant action in the gastrointestinal tract than the cruder ones. (4) Pure materials may be administered parenterally, whereas crude digitalis may not. Thus the pure digitalis materials have important characteristics of convenience which simplify therapy.

On the other hand, although statements to the contrary are made, no good evidence exists that any one digitalis material is superior to the others in its action on the heart. They are all qualitatively the same, and differ only quantitatively. The superior results which have been reported for specific drugs probably arise from the reporters' greater experience with the material they prefer. It is a well-established fact in medicine that experience with a particular drug increases the effectiveness a doctor may have with it.

There are a large number of digitalis materials. They represent various species of plants and various stages of extraction and purification, some of which are listed in the Materia Medica.

Diuretics

These drugs increase the rate of urine production and are used primarily for the relief of cardiac edema and hence are discussed here rather than in the section of urinary disturbances. Many cardiologists now feel that in terms of practical usefulness the diuretics are at least the equal of the digitalis glycosides in the treatment of the congestive failure of heart disease. The diuretics are outstandingly dependable. In congestive failure they almost always relieve symptoms. In patients in whom digitalis has ceased to be effective, the diuretics regularly provide the needed relief, and are usually the only drugs to which one can turn. Their action is so prompt that in advanced congestive failure one dose often provides more relief in a few hours than the most effective type of digitalization may give in as many days. They do not supersede digitalis, which has a different kind of action, but both may be combined for still greater effectiveness. The diuretics are used solely for the relief of congestive heart failure. Often the edema is obvious, but in many instances it is hidden, or occult. In both types the relief provided by a diuretic may be dramatic. Most of the present interest in these drugs centers around the mercurial diuretics, which are outstanding because of their dependability and potency, but the other diuretics listed and discussed are still often used and have special merits of their own.

The diuretics by one mechanism or another increase the rate of urine formation. They do not act on the heart. Large depots of edema may be seen to melt away during one night, a night during which the patient may pass as much as 10 liters (about 11 quarts) of urine. In cases of edema hidden in the pulmonary bed or the liver, a single injection of a diuretic may cause a large output of urine with marked improvement in the patient's condition. The relief of the symptoms of congestive failure after these drugs are used comes solely from the removal of fluid from water-logged tissues and organs which passes out of the body in the urine. In the normal person without edema, relatively little effect may be obtained from the diuretics.

The diuretics may be classified as follows: (1) water, (2) non-threshold substances; (3) acid-forming diuretics; (4) xanthines; (5) mercurials; (6) the exchange resins, a new and not yet well-established group of substances which may soon become important materials in the relief of edema; (7) carbonic anhydrase inhibitors.

Water: Water is a diuretic, a fact which has long been recognized by the physiologist, but has not yet been accepted by all internists. This apparent paradox occurs because water washes sodium out of the body, and sodium is the ion which binds water to the tissues. Thus the drinking of several quarts of water may wash away enough sodium to result in the liberation of bound water and to produce a diuresis. Excessive amounts of *tap* water may even produce symptoms of serious dehydration. It is for this reason that men working in the heat of steel mills and shipyards are required to take sodium chloride tablets every time they drink water. This procedure prevents the development of heat cramps (really due to sodium deficit), which were common in these industries when the men drank tap water. Tap water is the diuretic, saline or salt water is not.

It has already been pointed out that in the cardiac patient a disturbance exists which produces salt retention; in turn, the salt retention holds the water and forms the edema. It has been amply demonstrated by experiment and clinical experience that the administration of large amounts of water (of the order of 5 to 10 quarts daily) produces a diuresis and removes edema in patients. Nevertheless, a number of cardiologists still restrict water intake sharply. This precaution is necessary only when the salt intake is not carefully limited, but is unnecessary when salt is limited. Clinical experience and substantial physiologic considerations support the practice of permitting cardiac patients whose salt intake is restricted, to drink as much water as they wish, and to encourage the drinking of at least 1500 cc. (about 2 quarts) daily. It must be remembered that this applies only to tap water, and not to other fluids such as milk or some brands of carbonated beverage which contain sodium.

Nonthreshold Diuretics: These are materials which, when taken by mouth, are excreted almost quantitatively in the urine. They carry away water by their osmotic tension. This extra water is the diuresis they provide for the patient. Urea is the most common diuretic of this type. It is effective, but has a decidedly bad taste which is difficult to mask. It is relatively nontoxic. The doses are large, of the order of 15 Gm. daily, and, in terms of 0.5 Gm. capsules, total 30 per day, a quantity of capsules which many patients bluntly refuse to take. Urea is often taken in a 50 per cent solution of water. It is best tolerated when well chilled.

Acid-Forming Diuretics: As their name implies, these diuretics are sources of acid. To prevent the development of acidosis, the sodium of the tissues neutralizes the acid. The removal of sodium in this process liberates water formerly bound by the sodium. This water moves into the blood stream and thence into the urine. Unless there is neutralization and excretion of these drugs when they are used, acidosis may develop. In patients with renal insufficiency, acidosis may be a real danger. These drugs also frequently produce gastric distress, especially when the large doses, which are usually necessary, are used. There are some observers who feel that the acid-forming drugs may also cause renal irritation.

The acid-forming drugs are not very potent diuretics and can be counted on for satisfactory diuresis only in cases of mild congestive failure. However, they potentiate (increase) the effectiveness of the xanthine and mercurial diuretics and this is the purpose for which they are most frequently used today. The usual dose is of the order of 6 to 9 Gm. daily, divided into 3 doses. The tablets are 0.5 Gm. and are usually enteric coated to prevent gastric irritation. Some physicians give these drugs daily; others use a different schedule giving the acid-forming diuretics only for a day or two preceding and a day or two following each injection of a mercurial. Only one preparation, ammonium chloride is used today with any frequency.

Xanthine Diuretics: The xanthine diuretics are closely related to caffeine, chemically and pharmacologically. They all increase the rate of urine formation, presumably by increasing the rate of salt elimination by the kidney. Their effectiveness as diuretics is not outstanding. They also stimulate the cerebrum and produce excitement and insomnia. Caffeine is the most potent in these respects and for that reason is not used as a diuretic but is sometimes used for its stimulant action. The xanthine drugs also relax smooth muscle of the bronchi. There is evidence which is not convincing that they relax the smooth muscle of the coronary arteries. For this reason they are used in angina pectoris and coronary infarction, a practice far more common ten years ago than at present. Many cardiologists use these drugs only in cases of bronchial spasm and pulmonary edema.

The xanthine drugs are relatively insoluble; hence, they are sometimes mixed with other materials to increase solubility. Adequate doses frequently produce gastric distress. Attempts have been made to solve the problem of gastric distress by coating the tablets. In most instances, however, gastric distress is still their chief disadvantage in doses large enough to produce diuresis. When they can be used as diuretics, they have the advantage of oral administration. Commonly used preparations are listed in the Materia Medica.

Mercurial Diuretics: These drugs are the outstanding members of the diuretic group; they are the most dependable, the most effective and the most potent. They are widely used because of these qualities. A patient with advanced congestive failure, cyanotic, with a chest full of fluid, gasping for air and sitting upright because of orthopnea, may lose as much as 15 pounds of edema as the result of a single injection. Overnight the picture may change from a moribund patient to one who is comfortable, lies flat with no respiratory distress, and is anxious to get out of bed. Such dramatic changes are now commonplace. Most cardiologists feel that these are lifesaving and lifesparing drugs in congestive heart failure. On the other hand, because of their potency, the improper use of these drugs has led to some poor results and bad reactions. Some physicians feel that the mercurials are too potent to be used frequently, some reserve them only for the most serious cases, and some do not use them at all. Nevertheless, the use of the mercurial diuretics has been vastly increased in terms of medical indications, numbers of patients, and size and frequency of doses. Some physicians use them in all cases of congestive failure, no matter how mild.

Mode of action: All the mercurial diuretics act in the same way, by increasing the elimination of sodium by the kidney. As a result, the water that was bound by the sodium is also eliminated. It is important in this connection to note that the kidney must be able to form urine. The mercurial diuretic will not induce diuresis in a kidney which does not produce any urine at all. There must be water available and kidneys which function. This is usually the case in heart disease, and this is the condition in which a mercurial diuretic is most dependable. In renal disease, however, the mercurial is not always effective, a result which may be due to kidneys incapable of forming urine. Many cardiologists will not use the mercurial diuretics in renal disease, and virtually all are agreed that the mercurials are contraindicated in acute glomerular nephritis and the nephrosis of children.

Duration of effects: The diuretic action of the mercurial usually begins to develop in an hour or two after the injection and usually persists for from 6 to 12 hours. Elimination is complete in from 12 to 24 hours. For this reason daily injections may usually be given without danger of accumulation, which is thought to be greater in patients in whom the injection is not followed by a diuresis.

Untoward effects: The mercurial diuretics are irritant materials. Their injection must be made skillfully. A poor intravenous injection with leakage around the vein may produce a thrombophlebitis, local necrosis or at the very least, a great deal of pain. Most of the preparations are mixed with theophylline, which decreases their local irritant action. One preparation (mercaptomerin) is a combination with a thiol material which reduces local irritant action to such an extent that subcutaneous injection is permissible. The standard preparations are usually given intramuscularly, but one of them, meralluride, may also be given subcutaneously. The intravenous route is now used relatively rarely. Tablets for oral administration and rectal suppositories are effective but produce a large amount of local irritation and are rarely used.

It is not surprising that the mercurial diuretics should cause unpleasant reactions; they are potent drugs. A large number of reactions may be attributed to poorly administered injections. The intramuscular injections should be made deeply into the muscle, and not the gluteal fat, of the buttock. In order to insure an intramuscular injection the upper and outer quadrant of the buttock is chosen. The injection should be made well away from the mid-portion of the buttock. It is better technic to spread the skin tight around the point of injection instead of, as is more common, pinching the skin and injecting through the fold. The former method makes for a deeper injection and is less painful.

No matter how good the technic of the injection, cramps may soon develop in the muscle injected. They may last as long as 30 minutes, but rarely longer. Little can be done to ease the discomfort other than to have the patient rest. An injection which causes violent pain radiating down the leg has very likely been made around a nerve fiber. Such pain is always the result of poor technic. Involvement of the nerve fiber infrequently results in a serious or permanent neurologic complication.

Other disagreeable effects are usually from the systemic actions of these drugs. After a large diuresis patients often complain of cramps in the abdomen and the calves of the legs. The cramps may be due to the removal of large amounts of sodium and the production of a sodium deficit, giving rise to the development of symptoms akin to heat cramps. Weakness and nervousness may also result from the sodium deficit. Excessive dehydration with sodium deficit after the use of mercurial drugs in combination with rigid salt restriction for long periods of time has been reported. Such reactions must be watched for and avoided, and the doctor should be informed of the first evidences of it. Sometimes an examination of the blood for sodium will anticipate such a reaction. It may be suspected in all cases of persistent intense weakness, lassitude or prolonged cramps following the use of mercurials. These symptoms may be relieved by a dose of salt, but a dose of salt will also produce water retention; the decision to use the salt should, therefore, be made by the physician. It is better practice to give smaller doses of the diuretic and thereby avoid the distressing situation.

Other symptoms of an unwanted reaction in mercurial diuresis—skin rashes, fever, giddiness, fainting, palpitations and, rarely, death—may be due to sensitivity. Febrile reactions, which may come on an hour or two after a morning injection and then decline during the afternoon are often confused with infections and treated with penicillin instead of discontinuing the offending mercurial. Some patients have a highly specific hypersensitivity to one of the mercurials, but can use the others without reaction; in other cases the hypersensitivity extends to all the mercurials and the patient can take none of them.

The development of acute prostatism from excessive diuresis is a special complication presented by the elderly male. The prostatism may be accompanied by complete obstruction to the flow of urine and may add many new problems. This is yet another reason for moderation in the diuresis demanded of these drugs, but moderation does not imply ineffective doses.

Dosage: The usual dose of the mercurial diuretics (all are of approximately the same potency) is from 1 to 2 cc. In sensitive patients adequate diuresis may sometimes be obtained with 0.5 cc. or even 0.25 cc., but these cases are few. Rarely patients may for a time require 3 or 4 cc. daily to induce diuresis. The interval between injections varies. Many physicians administer the drug daily in selected cases. Others will not follow such a schedule. One of the most efficient plans is frequently and regularly to give the drug in doses which produce a moderate but not a massive diuresis until a "dry weight" is reached; then a new dosage and a new interval between doses are determined to maintain the effect. The term "dry weight" means the *ideal* weight of the patient, that is, the weight of the patient in a normal state of hydration with only the edema fluid removed; the term does not mean, as is sometimes misconstrued, a state of abnormal dehydration. The dose for maintenance is one which, determined by trial, does not produce excessive diuresis or disagreeable symptoms, but removes edema and maintains dry weight. Small doses given at frequent intervals are better than infrequent large doses followed by massive diuresis and disagreeable side effects.

The mercurial diuretics which are currently in use are listed in the Materia Medica.

Exchange Resins

These constitute a new group of drugs now being tested for

their practical value in the treatment of congestive failure. Since the effect of the exchange resins in congestive heart failure is to produce a diuresis, they are included here. In general they are of limited utility and only occasionally simplify matters for the cardiac patient.

The exchange resins are used to remove sodium from food. They were of great value during the late war as a material to make sea water potable for shipwrecked sailors by removing its salt. The proper exchange resin, when taken with a normally salted diet, will prevent the intestinal tract from absorbing the sodium. Thus a patient may be able to eat food he likes, prepared in a manner he prefers with respect to salt, and yet, as far as absorbed sodium is concerned, be on a salt-poor diet. Salt restriction makes the diet so unpalatable for some patients that the dietary relief permitted by the exchange resins provides a much-sought-for solution. The exchange resins have some disadvantages, however, chief among these being that the resins are not yet highly selective and remove potassium and calcium as well as the sodium. Thus potassium and calcium deficiencies have resulted from the use of exchange resins. It is to be hoped that the exchange resins can be made more selective so that their use will not be attended by the danger of serious potassium or calcium deficiencies. In the presently used preparations precautions have been taken to prevent these complications and, for the most part, they have proved to be effective. Another serious effect of the resins is the production of intractable constipation and even intestinal obstruction. The patient, must be carefully watched for the development of constipation when the resins are used regularly. Many patients object to the texture of the resins.

Carbonic Anhydrase Inhibitors: These are a new class of drugs which produce diuresis by interfering with the formation of carbonic acid in the blood. Acetazoleamide (diamox) is one of these presently being tested by the oral route. It seems to be effective, but more extensive trial is necessary for final evaluation.

Disorders of Cardiac Rhythm

The cardiac arrhythmias are common and disturbing developments in heart disease; sometimes they are of a very serious nature and the prompt and proper treatment may be a matter of vital importance to the patient. In some cases a cardiac arrhythmia is not particularly important and if the patient is given a sedative he may "sleep it off," but in other cases treatment is complex. Quinidine and procaine amide are the most important drugs used today for the relief of disturbances in cardiac rhythm.

Quinidine

This alkaloid is extracted along with quinine from the bark of the cinchona tree. It has the same chemical formula as quinine but has a somewhat different arrangement of atoms and is an optical isomer of quinine. Both quinidine and quinine have similar actions. They exert the same effect on the plasmodia of malaria, and are about equally potent. Quinine is used for malaria largely because it is much cheaper than quinidine, not because it is better. In the case of the cardiac actions, however, although both exert similar actions on the heart, quinidine is considerably more potent and can produce a degree of cardiac effect that cannot be duplicated by any dose of quinine.

Mode of action: The action of quinidine on heart muscle is one of depression: it depresses conduction in cardiac muscle, depresses the ability of the heart muscle to initiate its contractions and prolongs the refractoriness of cardiac muscle (that is, after a contraction it prolongs the period during which the heart will not respond to another stimulus). Quinidine does not improve the action of the myocardium per se. These actions of quinidine are useful in abolishing abnormal cardiac rhythms. It is useful in auricular fibrillation and flutter, premature contractions, auricular and nodal tachycardias, and ventricular tachycardia and fibrillation.

Administration: Quinidine is well absorbed from the gastrointestinal tract, its full effects developing in about 2 hours. The drug is usually taken orally in the form of the sulfate, a single dose being from 0.3 to 0.6 Gm. The interval between doses depends on the effects produced and desired. Recently, a preparation of quinidine sulfate dissolved in propylene glycol has become available for intramuscular injection. This is useful only in cases in which oral administration is not feasible. The dosage is the same as in the oral tablet, and the effects develop in about the same period of time.

Untoward effects: The use of quinidine in auricular fibrillation has resulted in accidents in which clots have been discharged from the auricles at the instant that the normal rhythm was restored and the auricles began to contract forcibly. The breaking away of a clot is not an action of the drug per se, but is a danger inherent in the abolition of auricular fibrillation, and is a result of the desired effect, namely, the restoration of contraction in auricles which for a period were not contracting. It is an accident which will happen with any drug used to restore normal rhythm in cases of auricular fibrillation. The decision for the doctor to make is not whether quinidine is safe but whether it is safe to restore a normal rhythm in a case of auricular fibrillation. This danger does not exist in other rhythmic disorders.

Some accidents have followed the use of quinidine in ventricular tachycardia, which is a rhythm so fraught with danger that any procedure, as well as the failure to act, may end in disaster. Regardless of possible accident, ventricular tachycardia must be slowed. Some drug must be used for this purpose, and quinidine is as safe as any other, including the newly available procaine amide.

Unpleasant side effects from quinidine are often called cinchonism and include buzzing in the ears, visual disturbances and giddiness.

Procaine Amide (Pronestyl)

This new addition to the drugs used in heart disease is presently used mainly for rhythmic disorders arising in the ventricle. The origin of procaine amide is interesting. It had been noted that procaine could be used to abolish disorders of cardiac rhythm in experimental animals. This observation was then applied to patients with normal hearts in whom disorders of cardiac rhythm developed during operation as the result of anesthesia. Procaine proved to be effective, but had the disadvantages of being short-lived and of requiring intravenous injection. Procaine amide has the same effect as procaine of which it is a derivative; however, procaine amide has a prolonged action and may be given both orally and parenterally. It has replaced procaine for correcting disorders of cardiac rhythm during anesthesia.

Experience has proved that procaine amide is effective in rhythmic disorders which develop in heart disease as well as during anesthesia. It is relatively ineffective in disturbances arising in the auricles but is successful in the abolition of ventricular premature contractions, ventricular tachycardia and ventricular fibrillation. The drug is given in single doses of 100 to 200 mg., the intervals between doses being determined by the effect produced. The route, oral or intravenous, is determined by the urgency of the case.

In the short period of time in which the drug has been on trial, there have been many successes and some failures. The dangers which are always present in ventricular tachycardia are still present when procaine amide is used to abolish it.

Cardiac Stimulants

Cardiac stimulation represents a hopeful kind of therapy; in an emergency, drugs in this category will stimulate the heart to perform while other failing organs in the body improve. These drugs are much to be desired, but whether such effects are obtainable is questionable. For this purpose such drugs as nikethamide (coramine) and pentylenetetrazole (metrazol) are now used. The dangers of adrenalin have already been discussed. Formerly, caffeine, camphor and strychnine were used for this purpose.

Recently two drugs closely related to epinephrine, arterenol (nor-epinephrine) and isopropyl arterenol (isopropyl nor-epinephrine) have provided new facets of epinephrine actions. These drugs represent a separation of the major epinephrine actions; arterenol, the action on the blood vessels and isopropyl arterenol, the epinephrine action directly on the heart. The latter preparation may, therefore, be used for direct stimulation of the heart without calling into action the pressor effects of epinephrine which by intense constriction of the arterial bed, may increase the burden on the heart.

Rheumatic Fever

Rheumatic fever is a disease of young people which characteristically causes exquisitely painful and swollen joints and frequently also seriously damages the heart. Treatment, therefore, is directed toward the prevention of heart disease as well as against the painful joints.

Salicylates

Their position in the treatment of heart disease is not settled. Salicylates are used in large amounts in the treatment of rheumatic fever. For the most part it is agreed that their function is merely to relieve the pain and the swelling of the joints. On the other hand there are some cardiologists who feel that they also protect the heart against the typical injuries of rheumatic fever and advise that large doses be used for this purpose. This view, however, is not held by most cardiologists.

Sodium salicylate is the salicylate drug most commonly prescribed, although acetylsalicylic acid (aspirin) may also be used. The doses are large, of the order of a total of 6 to 7 Gm. daily, given in about 6 doses. Such doses often cause intestinal irritation with nausea and cramps, as well as dizziness and buzzing in the ears. Sodium bicarbonate is sometimes given to relieve these symptoms, but the evidence is that sodium bicarbonate hastens the elimination of salicylates. The same effect, therefore, may be obtained by giving smaller doses of the salicylates.

In instances in which extremely large doses of salicylates are prescribed for their specific effect on the heart itself, parenteral administration may sometimes be used; but usually the material is given orally. The effects come on in about 30 minutes and last about 4 hours, depending on the size of the dose. When high blood levels of the salicylates are sought and exceptionally large doses are used, the precaution of chemical determinations of the blood salicylate concentration must be taken. In such cases, if there is poisoning, collapse may occcur.

Cortisone and Corticotropin (ACTH)

It is hard to put drugs like cortisone (cortone, compound E) and corticotropin (ACTH) into a proper category at this time, because their mode of action is not yet precisely defined. They are also discussed in the section on endocrine disorders (page 212). Cortisone is a hormonal material extracted from the adrenal gland; corticotropin, a hormonal material extracted from the pituitary gland, stimulates the adrenal gland to produce cortisone. Thus both produce similar results. Their effects are principally on the mesenchymal tissue system, that is, the connective tissues of the body, and they are useful in cardiovascular disease in those conditions— the so-called collagen diseases—which are related to this tissue system. These diseases include rheumatic fever, lupus erythematosus and periarteritis nodosa. Whether cortisone or corticotropin provides a cure for any of these diseases, or only relief, is still to be determined. It is of outstanding importance, however, that specific agents have finally been found for a group of serious cardiovascular diseases which were heretofore without specific or even helpful medication.

The effects of these drugs in rheumatic fever are dramatic. Discomforts disappear in the first few days, the child looks well, and a sense of well-being quickly replaces the illness, depression, and exhaustion. Pain and swelling vanish, and the laboratory indexes of active disease quickly return to normal. The patient seems better, improves in color and gains weight. During the administration of these drugs,damage to the heart rarely develops and heart injuries already present seem to get better. When the laboratory evidence is definite that the active process has disappeared, the drug can be discontinued. Whether there will be a relapse cannot be predicted, and it may be necessary in some cases to repeat the treatment.

Hypertension

Hypertension is a serious and disabling cardiovascular condition. The cause of this condition is not known and many of the mechanisms in its development are still obscure. It is presently thought, that for reasons still unknown, the smaller arteries or arterioles in the body tend to narrow or constrict, and, in order for sufficient blood to get through, the heart has to pump at a higher pressure than normally. Most modern treatments are directed against the increased tone in the arterioles and attempt to reduce it by one means or another.

Many forms of treatment for hypertension have been tried and many more are presently under experimental observation, for this is still one of our serious and entirely inadequately treated medical problems. Of the forms of treatment already tried, it may be categorically stated that there is no one form which is entirely or uniformly satisfactory. There have been many diets devised but their effects, at best, are temporary. There are many forms of medication of questionable utility. New forms of medication get into the newspapers daily, and in general, most of these have serious inherent dangers. There are operations to reduce blood pressure, and while these are sometimes the only effective measures, they still leave much to be desired. Most of the best medical treatments are directed against the symptoms rather than the disease itself. Some of the drugs which are occasionally still used in an attempt to reduce blood pressure are briefly described below.

Sympathetic blockaders (see page 119) have been used in the treatment of hypertension with the hope that they might provide a pharmacologic sympathetcomy and produce results comparable to surgical sympathectomy. Such effects from these drugs, however, are short-lived and generally disappointing. At the time of this writing a member of this group of drugs, hexamethonium derivatives are being widely tried in the treatment of hypertension. Earlier experiences in England and some experiences already gathered here, indicate that these are also toxic drugs, to be used only with the greatest caution. There is the additional experience with these drugs, that when a satisfactory effect is produced there is a tendency for the patient to develop tolerance to the drug, so that even in these cases, the drug is soon useless.

Blood Clotting

Intravascular blood clots may give rise to serious and even fatal embolism in patients with coronary infarctions. Similarly, in rheumatic heart disease with mitral stenosis and all heart disease in which there is auricular fibrillation, there is danger of clot formation and embolization. In thrombophlebitis clots form in the inflamed veins, and these may break off into the bloodstream and cause pulmonary embolism. In all these conditions the tendency to formation of clots and to the propagation of clots already formed may be depressed by the use of anticoagulant drugs, discussed in some detail in the chapter on blood.

There are two types of anticoagulants: heparin which produces immediate effects, and the dicumarol drugs whose effects take about

24 hours to develop fully. Each, therefore, has its special indication.

It may be noted that the depression of the clotting mechanism by any of these drugs may lead to serious hemorrhage from cuts and wounds, and even serious internal hemorrhage without injury. When these drugs are used, the patient and his clotting mechanism must be carefully watched by regular tests in order to determine and limit the extent of drug action. When the limit of safe action has been exceeded, the effects can be reversed by blood transfusion in the case of heparin or the injection of vitamin K in the case of dicumarol.

Shock

Shock is a vascular disorder in which the fundamental disturbance is a loss of tone and dilatation of the capillary bed. This may develop as the result of trauma, hemorrhage, serious infection, burns, or intoxication. As a consequence of this widening of the vascular bed, the resistance to the flow of blood is reduced so greatly that blood pressure falls markedly. The vascular bed is so enlarged that the blood normally in the body is insufficient in amount to fill it. Because of these two effects, the transfer of essential elements between the blood and cells is so inefficient that if permitted to continue for a substantial period irreversible tissue damage develops. This is a most discouraging experience which is sometimes encountered in a case of shock. The shock is finally overcome with plasma infusions and the patient appears to be making a good recovery, but he goes abruptly into a decline and dies of kidney insufficiency. The reason, of course, is that these organs were permanently injured by the too long continued shock. Shock is one of the grave emergencies in medicine and it must be quickly reversed if life is to be saved.

The most important aspect of treatment of shock is to increase the volume of fluid in the bloodstream; this not only increases blood pressure but also favors vital cellular exchange. The best material for this purpose is whole blood or plasma. These should be used in amounts necessary to restore the blood pressure to an effective level. Epinephrine (adrenalin) may produce deleterious effects even though it may temporarily elevate the blood pressure. Its action is to constrict the arterioles to such a marked degree that even though it produces a rise in blood pressure there may actually be a diminution in the amount of blood which is able to circulate through the vascular system and reach the capillary bed where it is vitally needed. On the other hand, when properly controlled, this type of epinephrine action may be a life-saving measure in some cases of shock. A similar effect, with fewer difficulties may be obtained from the use of arterenol or from other sympathomimetic amines.

Other Drugs Used in Heart Disease

Blood plasma and blood substitutes are sometimes needed in the acute stages of cardiac disease in which circulatory shock has developed. In heart disease complicated by this serious condition, fluid may not be given as freely or as rapidly as it is in the noncardiac patient. Indeed, some physicians never use plasma even when shock develops in the cardiac patient. They are afraid that the additional fluid in the circulation may overburden the heart. The patient's blood pressure must be carefully watched, and the lungs must be frequently observed for the development of pulmonary edema when plasma is administered.

Oxygen is often given to patients with cardiac emergencies. It is used in cases in which shock, pulmonary embolism, pulmonary edema, pleural effusion, ventricular tachycardia, or other cardiac complications cause insufficient oxygenation of the blood. It has no direct action on the heart. The inhalation of higher concentrations of oxygen than is normally present in air may increase the amount of oxygen which dissolves in blood. In some cases this may relieve cyanosis and dyspnea. The oxygen provides relief, but it does not cure; at best, oxygen offers symptomatic relief. On the other hand, it is never harmful.

Varicose Veins

Varicose veins are a great burden to many people, causing swelling of the legs and extensive skin damage. They occur most frequently in females who have borne many children and in men whose occupations keep them on their feet a great deal of the time. The only way to cure this condition is by removing the defective veins. While this may be done surgically, it may also be done pharmacologically. That is to say, drugs called sclerotics may be used to irritate the internal lining of the veins to the extent that thromboses develop, and these, in turn, obilterate the veins. Unfortunately, the most common sequel is, that some time after the effects of the varicose veins on the skin have cleared up and the condition seems cured, the thromboses are canalized, blood again flows through them, and the original condition returns. A combination of a small operation in which the vein is tied off from above so that the blood cannot run back into it and the use of the sclerosing drugs, often results in a complete cure. Hemorrhoids are varicose veins of the rectal region and in some cases may be treated by sclerotic agents.

Capillary Fragility

Capillary fragility may increase as the result of anoxemia of some duration, intoxications and entirely unknown causes. The net result is that fluid filters out of the capillary bed too easily and is not well reabsorbed. This is so principally because osmotic pressure which draws fluid toward the capillaries diminishes in potency when the capillary membrane is damaged. This results in edema and interferes with the exchange of gases, electrolyte and metabolites between blood and cells. The repair of such damage is essential to life; usually this is difficult, sometimes impossible. Oxygen, vitamin C (ascorbic acid) and rutin are used in an attempt to restore capillary integrity.

Spasm of Blood Vessels

Spasm of branches of the coronary arteries which occurs in angina pectoris, vasospastic disease and spasm secondary to thrombosis and embolism requires the action of a vasodilator drug to relax or dilate the blood vessels. We have seen, in the section on anginal pain, that nitrites are the most important group of drugs used to relax spasm of the coronary arteries, that they are both effective and dependable. Unfortunately, the situation is quite different in the case of vasospastic disease and vasospasm due to thrombosis and embolism; arterial spasm in these conditions is usually entirely unresponsive to the nitrites.

As the result of plugging a blood vessel in a case of thrombophlebitis or in arterial embolism, there may be intense spasm of the blood vessel. This reflex phenomenon makes matters worse since it considerably increases the difficulty blood has in getting through the involved blood vessel. It is for this reason that vasodilatation is therapeutically useful. The most certain way of obtaining vasodilatation is by blocking the nerves involved and abolishing the reflex. In the case of embolism of an artery in the lower extremities this may be relatively simply accomplished; sacral block or even low spinal anesthesia may be applied. Heat sometimes induces vasodilatation. There is also a fairly long list of drugs which are used for this purpose, papaverine, being the oldest, and the newer sympathetic blockaders such as tolazoline (priscoline) being the most recent. The theoretic advantages of these drugs are not often of practical value and only rarely are these drugs of real help.

Vasospastic disturbances, such as Raynaud's disease, are often functional conditions with a large psychogenic element. The effect of vasodilators in these conditions is, at best, only temporary. It may also be categorically stated that these drugs are of no value in arteriosclerosis and in thromboangiitis obliterans (Buerger's disease) in which they are occasionally also used.

Vasodilators

Papaverine is a material extracted from the poppy and used to dilate arteries. It is used almost exclusively in cases of arterial embolism to cause dilatation of the plugged vessels in order to permit the blood to flow around the clot. In some cases papaverine has been very effective in this regard, but to a large extent the new sympatholytic drugs such as tolazoline (priscoline) have been found more effective and have replaced it.

Depropanex, an extract of pancreatic tissue, produces vasodilatation. It is used exclusively to relieve vasospasm in arterial disease of the extremities. In intermittent claudication, injections or oral doses of this material have occasionally seemed to produce good results. Patients with impending gangrene due to endarteritis have been benefited by it. On the other hand, in a large number of cases such desirable effects have not occurred.

Nicotinic acid (niacin) is used to produce vasodilatation. This agent is the effective vitamin fraction in nicotinamide, differing in action only in that it also produces cutaneous vasodilatation. Many patients who once took nicotinic acid for its vitamin action were surprised to discover that it also made them flush. The amide of nicotinic acid (nicotinamide) does not have the flushing action. It is not certain that the flush is more than skin deep in cases in which nicotinic acid is used to produce vasodilatation.

Posterior pituitary extract and the purified pitressin have vasopressor actions. Because of a direct effect on the smooth muscle of the intestine and the arteries, they produce many disagreeable side effects, present real dangers, and are rarely used to elevate the blood pressure in the cardiac patient.

Autonomic Drugs

These drugs act on the autonomic nervous system (the sympathetic and the parasympathetic nervous systems), on various organs throughout the body, on the heart and blood vessels. Their effects on the cardiovascular system are sometimes very dramatic but they are not drugs of the first importance in heart disease. Although they are also discussed elsewhere they will be briefly considered here in relation to their cardiovascular actions.

Sympathomimetic Drugs

These are related in action and structure to epinephrine (adrenlin). They mimic the action of stimulation of the sympathetic nervous system, accelerate the heart, increase the blood pressure and heighten the tone of the arterioles (that is, constrict them). Their use in heart disease is limited, but they may be extremely helpful in heart block with frequent Adams-Stokes episodes or with a ventricular rate that is too slow.

An injection of epinephrine directly into a heart that has stopped as a terminal event in the course of some fatal noncardiac disease, sometimes makes it beat again. This dramatic gesture is often tried, but is almost never of any real value. Sometimes the heart takes a few extra beats, but it never continues for long. Epinephrine has value in noncardiac conditions such as some types of poisoning, anaphylactic shock and primary shock.

Some dangers which may attend the use of the sympathomimetic drugs in heart disease should be considered when any of these drugs are used for purposes such as the common practice of instilling them in the nose for nasal decongestion in colds. Epinephrine and similar drugs increase the work of the heart, which may be undesirable in some forms of heart disease. In hypertension the blood pressure may climb to dangerous levels. In coronary artery disease, the arterioles may constrict, further diminishing the blood supply to the myocardium, or the sudden elevation in blood pressure may cause a rupture of the ventricle in case of a ventricular infarct. An attack of pulmonary edema may be mistaken for an attack of bronchial asthma, and while epinephrine may help the asthma, in the case of pulmonary edema it may make matters worse. In the treatment of heart disease, epinephrine should be reserved for patients in whom the indications have been defined by the attending physician and should be used according to the orders left by him. It should not be used indiscriminately whenever collapse occurs or the pulse is not easily palpated.

A long list of drugs belong to this group, all related to epinephrine, pharmacologically and chemically. Ephedrine is used mainly in heart block and orthostatic hypotension; it is given orally. Hydroxyamphetamine may be used in shock to elevate blood pressure. Methamphetamine has much the same action as amphetamine (benzedrine) which is used mostly for its central stimulant action. It is, however, effective in orthostatic hypotension, elevating the blood pressure and producing a sense of good feeling. Phenylephrine (neosynephrine) is a powerful vasoconstrictor and elevates the blood pressure. While it has useful local actions, the interest of the cardiologist is in its effectiveness in raising blood pressure in shock. Many other agents in this group have similar actions, but for the most part their use is limited to that of nasal decongestion.

As already mentioned there are now available two drugs closely related to epinephrine which seem to represent a separation of the two primary actions of epinephrine: arterenol (nor-epinephrine) and isopropyl arterenol (isopropyl nor-epinephrine). Arterenol exhibits mainly the action of epinephrine on the arterioles to constrict them and raise blood pressure; this action, however, is more long-lived than with epinephrine. Isopropyl arterenol has the direct action of epinephrine to stimulate the heart and the antiallergic action of epinephrine.

Arterenol may be used, therefore, for its vascular actions without appreciable stimulation of the heart, an effect which may be especially useful in shock following coronary infarction, in which the direct action of epinephrine may lead to cardiac arrhymias. Isopropyl arterenol may be used for its direct stimulatory effect on the heart, in heart block, or for its antiallergic effect in asthma, without elevating the blood pressure.

Sympatholytic Drugs

The sympatholytic drugs have interesting actions on the cardiovascular system. Each one of the sympatholytic drugs differs slightly from the others, but in general, they have similar actions, blocking the typical sympathomimetic effects of epinephrine, or the stimulation of the adrenal glands or the sympathetic nerves. These drugs include benzodioxane, tolazoline, and tetraethylammonium (TEA). By their sympatholytic action they lower blood pressure and relieve vasospasm. For this reason they may be used in vasospastic diseases (such as Raynaud's disease); in embolism, they dilate arteries and permit blood to pass around the embolus. Tolazoline is used perhaps more than the others for the latter purpose. These drugs can be counted on for temporary relief only; their depressant effects in high blood pressure are short-lived, attended by dangers, and in general very disappointing.

An outstanding use of these drugs is in testing for the presence of pheochromocytoma, a tumor of the adrenal gland, which forms excessive amounts of adrenalin and produces episodes of marked elevation of blood pressure. This effect of the excess adrenalin can be counteracted by a dose of benzodioxane, and forms the basis for the test. In addition, during the operation for the removal of the tumor, special hazards are associated with the outpouring of large amounts of adrenalin into the blood stream, and benzodioxane may be used during the operation to protect against them.

At this time, these drugs are of greater interest in the laboratory and as research material than for their practical value. It is to be hoped that some derivative will be synthesized which will have greater practical usefulness.

Parasympathomimetic Drugs

These drugs slow the heart, lower blood pressure and have other extracardiac effects. These actions are only rarely useful in the treatment of heart disease. Occasionally, in such rhythmic disorders as sinus and auricular tachycardias, a dose of methacholine (mecholyl) terminates the aberrant rhythm. An injection of 25 mg., which is the usual dose, also has many unpleasant side effects such as intense nausea, vomiting and a sense of oppression in the chest. The antidote for this effect, if it is too intense, is atropine (2 mg.) by hypodermic injection. This dose should be kept ready in a sterile syringe whenever it is used. Methacholine may also precipitate an asthmatic attack. Other parasympathomimetic drugs, such as neostigmine and other choline derivatives, are not used for their effects on the cardiovascular system.

Parasympatholytic Drugs

Atropine antagonizes the action of methacholine, paralyzes the vagus nerve, and accelerates the heart. Its use in cardiac disease is limited to its action as·an antidote when methacholine is used to abolish a rhythmic disorder and produces disagreeable effects. This group of drugs has no other uses in cardiovascular disease.

Drugs Used in Treatment of Cardiovascular Disease

Antibiotics	Hormones
Anticoagulants	Hypertensives
Autonomics	Sclerotics
Chemotherapeutics	Stimulants (heart muscle)
Depressants (heart muscle)	Vasoconstrictors
Diuretics	Vasodilators

Study Questions

1. Review the anatomy and physiology of the cardiovascular system.

2. By what means does the edema of congestive heart failure develop?

3. Why may morphine be contraindicated in patients who experience severe pain from cardiac disease such as infarction?

4. How do the effects of nitrites differ in normal individuals in contrast to those suffering from angina pectoris?

5. Contrast the values and disadvantages of amyl nitrite and nitroglycerin as used in the treatment of angina pectoris.

6. In what ways do the various digitalis materials differ from each other?

7. What are the two major beneficial actions of digitalis upon the heart? What indirect effects do these produce in the presence of heart failure?

8. What are the chief toxic effects of digitalis and what are the nurse's responsibilities in relation to these effects?

9. What are the uses of digitalis?

10. Nausea and vomiting may be toxic signs of digitalis. Of what factors should the nurse be aware in relation to these specific symptoms when caring for a patient receiving a digitalis preparation?

11. What knowledge should the nurse be aware of in relation to absorption and elimination of digitalis, schedules of administration, methods of administration?

12. How are digitalis materials standardized?

13. What is the relationship between digitalization dosages and maintenance doses of digitalis materials? Why are such differences necessary?

14. What advantages do purified forms of digitalis have over the crude forms?

15. For what purpose are diuretics administered?

16. In what ways may water, urea, acid forming salts, xanthines and mercurials act as diuretics?

17. Under what special conditions are mercurial diuretics especially useful? When are they contraindicated?

18. Ideally, at what time of day is it advisable to administer a diuretic such as one of the mercurial preparations? Why?

19. What special precautions should be taken in the parenteral administration of such a diuretic?

20. What is the mechanism of action of the exchange resins? Why may they be of especial value in the treatment of the cardiac patient?

21. What is the specific effect of procaine amide? Indicate its special uses.

22. What are the source, action, methods of administration, toxic symptoms, and uses of quinidine?

23. Review the actions and uses of the autonomic system drugs in relation to the cardiovascular system. Give examples.

24. In the treatment of shock, what is the most important objective of the medical treatment? How is this usually accomplished?

25. What is the method of action of sclerosing agents in the treatment of varicose veins?

26. Hyaluronidase is an enzyme which may be used for what purpose?

27. For what clinical conditions are vasodilators used? By what mechanisms are their actions brought about?

15

TREATMENT OF DIGESTIVE DISORDERS

The digestive system is made up of the hollow muscular organs, esophagus, stomach, small intestine, large intestine and rectum, through which food passes during the digestive process. There are also several accessory organs of the digestive system, the salivary glands, liver and gall-bladder, and pancreas; these supply digestive juices and digestive enzymes. The appendix, an organ with an uncertain function, also forms a part of the system.

The greater part of digestion and absorption takes place in the upper part of the tract, the stomach and small intestine; in the large intestine and rectum, water is absorbed, and the fecal mass assumes its final semi-solid form. The digestive juices consist of (1) saliva from the salivary glands, (2) hydrochloric acid and pepsin from the stomach, (3) bile from the liver and gallbladder, (4) pancreatic juice and (5) succus entericus from the small intestine. The intestinal contents are pushed along the digestive canal by a series of snake-like contractions or peristaltic waves.

The integrity and activity of the intestine and the character and amount of the digestive juices and enzymes determine the efficiency of the digestive process and the symptoms which may arise from any abnormality in the system. Thus, there may be symptoms due to congenital or mechanical defects in the stomach or intestine, irritation or injury to the lining of the alimentary tract, abnormal peristaltic activity, excessive or deficient formation or supply of digestive juices, poor food, poisoning, infections or infestations by worms or parasites. The common symptoms which may arise as a result of these disturbances are loss of appetite,

191

nausea, vomiting, pain, diarrhea, constipation, bloating, loss of weight and intestinal hemorrhage.

To a large extent the gastro-intestinal system, its motility as well as the production of digestive juices, is under the control of hormones and the autonomic nervous system which can stimulate or depress digestive function and intestinal activity.

Carbohydrate digestion takes place to a very limited extent in the mouth through the action of the saliva. In the stomach pepsin and hydrochloric acid begin more important digestive processes. The major portion of digestion, especially of protein and fats, occurs in the small intestine through the action of bile, pancreatic juice and the enzymes of the small intestine. Absorption of virtually all protein and fat also occurs in the small intestine. The large intestine is concerned mainly with the removal of water and electrolyte from the fecal mass which is in a fluid form when it leaves the small intestine.

Stimulants

Stimulation of intestinal motility and digestive juice formation can be brought about by autonomic drugs (such as methacholine, prostigmine) which mimic the effect of vagal stimulation. Irritation of one type or another may also stimulate intestinal activity and cause catharsis or diarrhea.

Cathartics

Cathartics, purgatives, physics, evacuants, and so forth differ only in the intensity of their effect on the bowel, but the effect itself is more or less the same: the bowel is evacuated by distending or irritating it. Most of these methods and drugs prevent the reabsorption of water in the large bowel or increase intestinal bulk either through an unabsorbed residue or by materials which swell on contact with water and by distending the colon promote peristaltic activity and the propulsion of the fecal mass toward the rectum. There are several classes of cathartics but they all have the same general disadvantages; if given in large doses all of them tend to produce griping, and given regularly they all favor habituation. There are some individual differences and it is usually wise to recognize a patient's preference for one cathartic over another. Since cathartics are often taken without medical advice, the patient usually has had previous experience with them and often has found the best one for himself by trial.

It is not wise to encourage the use of these drugs. Emphasis is often put on evacuation to the degree that a regular bowel movement may become a matter of vital psychic importance for a patient. This is not often the true state of physiologic affairs, for frequent bowel movements are not necessary as often as most people may think. Cathartics should be used only when there is a specific indication for their need or by order of the physician. Their regular use may lead to habituation and by decreasing muscle tone to chronic constipation.

Digestives

Digestives are materials which assist digestion either by replacing deficient digestive enzymes or juices, or by promoting their production. In general, drugs only act as digestives when they are needed to replace natural digestive materials which are lacking, for example, in cases in which bile or gastric acid is lacking, bile salts or hydrochloric acid may be effectively used as digestives.

Enzymes

Enzymes obtained from the organs of cattle, are used to replace digestive enzymes in cases in which there is reason to believe that the body does not produce them in sufficient quantity. These are little used today because of their dubious value. On the other hand, digestive enzymes are used in cooking to produce such pre-digested materials as junket, which is often well tolerated by patients with delicate digestive systems.

Bitters and Appetizers

Bitters and appetizers are materials which produce psychic stimulation of digestive juices because of their taste and aroma.

Acid

Acid, specifically hydrochloric acid, is used to replace normal gastric hydrochloric acid in certain cases, like pernicious anemia and achlorhydria, in which it is deficient in amount or entirely absent.

Choleretics and Cholegogues

Choleretics and cholegogues are drugs which stimulate the liver to produce bile and the gallbladder to empty its contents into the intestinal tract. Obviously, in cases in which a gallstone is blocking the passage of bile down the common bile duct, this type of drug action cannot be effective. The drugs used in this condition, because of their chemical nature, usually also aid directly in the digestive process, principally that of fat.

Emetics

Emetics are drugs which induce vomiting, either by irritating the intestinal tract or by a direct action on the brain. They are used principally in the treatment of poisoning. An overdosage of the locally acting emetics may produce serious damage to the stomach and small intestine. The only drug used to induce vomiting by a direct action on the brain is apomorphine.

Depressants

Depressants of intestinal activity are often needed to reduce the production of gastric juice, to relax intestinal spasm, to relieve vomiting and to relieve diarrhea. To some degree such effects can be produced by drugs which decrease the activity of the stomach by a vagolytic action, such as that produced by atropine or belladonna. This type of action is often accompanied by such disagreeable side effects as dryness of the mouth, dilatation of the pupils and difficulty in focusing on nearby objects. This is the reason for the search for drugs with a more intense action on the intestine and without much action elsewhere in the body. There are a number of atropine derivatives which have been introduced as substitutes because they were supposed to have this advantage over atropine. To date, most of these have not lived up to this promise; perhaps the only ones which are effective on the intestine other than atropine are methantheline (banthine) and diphenmethanil (prantal), both relatively new drugs.

Distention

Distention of the stomach and intestine with gas may be a most disagreeable condition. In many instances air swallowing is in a large part the cause of these accumulations of gas, and the best relief is provided by a correction of eating and breathing habits. In some cases, however, no such cause can be found, and intestinal stasis may play a role. Relief from distention is provided by any means which accelerates the liberation of the gas. Sometimes a small amount of drug which effervesces when it reaches the stomach gives the gas a much needed push. In cases of stasis the intestinal activity may be stimulated with a cathartic or a cholinergic drug. In acute conditions a stomach tube may relieve distention. Sometimes other physical methods, such as heat applied to the abdomen or use of a rectal tube, offer the simplest or most direct solutions to the problem.

Antacids

Antacids are drugs which inactivate the hydrochloric acid in the stomach by physical or chemical means. In general, these are alkaline materials, many with a buffering action, which combine with or neutralize stomach acid. They are used to reduce the amount of acid in the stomach which may be present in normally healthy people, or in patients with ulcers. In the former case the antacids are used to relieve "heart burn" or "water-brash." In the latter case antacids are used to remove the acid of the stomach which causes pain when it comes in contact with the ulcer.

A very important feature of antacids, especially the more potent ones, is what is called "rebound acidity," namely, the production of excess amounts of acid after the effects of the antacid have worn off. As a consequence of this effect, periods of great distress may set in after antacids have relieved pain or distress. The newer antacids, because they are largely buffering agents whose action is gentle and slow, tend to produce less rebound acidity than the simple alkalis.

One of the great dangers of two of the frequently used buffering materials, aluminum hydroxide gel and silica gels, is that they may cause serious obstipation or even intestinal obstruction when given in large amounts to patients who tend toward constipation.

This action may be due to the fact that they are clay-like nonabsorbable materials. The statement is made that some of the earthy antacid materials such as kaolin and the silicates, absorb toxic materials from the intestine in addition to their acid buffering action. This attractive notion, however, is far from a proved fact.

Exchange resins are still another group of new materials introduced for antacid action. They act by exchanging their own alkali for acid and have certain theoretically attractive features, including that of reduced rebound action. They are available alone or in mixtures containing buffering materials. The disadvantage of the resins lies in their unpleasant texture along with the tendency to produce serious constipation. The exchange resins are discussed in greater detail in another section when we consider the matter of how, in another form, they are used to remove sodium (page 173) in patients with heart failure.

Sedatives

Sedatives, often barbiturates, are frequently used in cases of overactivity of the intestinal tract. While such sedatives have no direct action on the intestinal tract, they not only tend to reduce intestinal activity but also allay the patient's distress by a sedative action on the brain. This is not surprising inasmuch as many intestinal symptoms are psychogenic in origin.

Antispasmodics

Antispasmodics are drugs used to relieve intestinal spasm. Such an effect may sometimes be obtained by local action with a demulcent, but more frequently a drug with a systemic action is used. In general, the same drugs that are used to depress intestinal activity are also used to relieve spasm. These are the vagolytic drugs such as atropine, belladonna and the more recent substitutes.

Antiseptics

Antiseptics were formerly used for a local action against bacteria in the intestine, but without much satisfactory effect. Since the chemical antiseptics which can kill intestinal bacteria were often almost as toxic to patients, their use has rightly been discontinued.

Today, however, intestinal antisepsis can easily be achieved by using the sulfa drugs and antibiotics. Most of the dysenteries are treated in this way. Also, they are often used preliminary to intestinal surgery to prevent peritoneal infection.

An interesting point concerning the antibiotics when they are used for long periods of time in the treatment of other diseases, is that they may produce an uncalled for degree of depression of normal intestinal flora with special symptoms resulting from it. Some types of bacterial action in the intestinal tract serve a useful purpose and symptoms may result from prolonged intestinal sterility. In addition, the antibiotics may not destroy all intestinal bacteria, and in that way favor the growth of varieties which are normally pushed into the background. One of the sources of difficulty with the broad-spectrum antibiotics is that they favor the development of *Monilia* by such a process. This infection, or so-called superinfection, rare under ordinary circumstances because the normal bacteria of the intestine prevent *Monilia* from growing, may cause anal and vulvar rashes with intense itching.

Vermifuges

Vermifuges are used in the treatment of worms and other intestinal parasites. Worm infestations are very common in some parts of this country. The types of worms vary and different remedies may be necessary for each type. It must be borne in mind that most of the drugs used for this purpose are toxic to higher forms of life than bacteria and tend to be hazardous to the patient. For this reason they must be used with care and discretion.

In many instances serious intoxication may result unless the patient can be made to evacuate promptly after the drug has acted. With some of the vermifuges special susceptibility is found in patients who are alcoholics. Some of the vermifuges are relatively more toxic after fatty meals because this leads to their absorption. Such food should, therefore, be avoided before taking these drugs.

There are other intestinal parasitic diseases, the most important of which is amebic dysentery. The treatment of this chronic and serious infection is a difficult one. But the problem has been simplified somewhat by a few of the now available specific remedies. These include the tetracyclines and some chemotherapeutic agents:

Ulcers

Ulcers are common and troublesome. The predominant symptom is pain. Some patients may lose weight, but in other cases the patient may discover that certain foods, such as milk relieve the pain, and as a consequence, these patients may gain a great deal of weight. Another symptom sometimes encountered is pain and burning on urination. This is not caused by the ulcer at all, but by the large amounts of strong alkalai medication that so many of these patients take to relieve the abdominal pain. The most serious problems in the treatment of ulcer are (1) resistance to treatment, (2) recurrence, (3) hemorrhage, (4) intestinal obstruction.

Most cases of ulcer respond readily to treatment. That is to say, in most cases the pain can be relieved by one or another of the antacids. Food and ulcer diets are also usually effective and in most instances the pain is soon relieved. There are, however, resistant cases in which none of the usual measures relieve the pain. When this is the case and the diagnosis is certain, surgery may provide the only answer to the problem.

The patient with the ulcer seems to have a constitutional disease; one which represents a particular kind of weakness. Many feel that in a large part peptic ulcers are psychosomatic conditions closely related to the worries and tensions of living, and that these as well as the ulcer itself require treatment if the patient is to be permanently cured. The vast majority of patients who are relieved by medical treatment and a large proportion of those who have had surgery, sooner or later suffer a recurrence of the ulcer.

In some cases the ulcer penetrates a large artery and causes serious intestinal hemorrhage. Treatment is either medical or surgical; the decision has to be made at the bedside.

Intestinal obstruction is another complication in patients who are apparently cured of their ulcers by medication. In this case the healed scar contracts and prevents the pasage of food through the duodenum. Surgery is usually the only recourse in this situation.

Diagnostic Drugs

Diagnostic drugs are frequently used in intestinal disease because the intestinal tract cannot be seen directly and much of diagnosis is made by test and by inference. The list of tests is a long one and involves the use of many special drugs (page 269). These tests include x-rays, gastric function tests, liver function tests, gallbladder function tests, stool analyses, test meals and blood tests for the absorption into the blood of digestive enzymes.

Drugs Used in Treatment of Digestive Disorders

Antacids	Cathartics
Antibiotics	Chemotherapeutics
Antiseptics (intestinal)	Choleretics
Antidiarrheals	Digestants
Antispasmodics	Emetics
Carminatives	Sialogogues

Study Questions

1. Review the anatomy and physiology of the gastro-intestinal tract.

2. What are the mechanisms of action of the various groups of cathartics?

3. What are the nurse's responsibilities in the administration of cathartics and the teaching of patients regarding their use?

4. What are special hazards encountered in the use of emetics, both local and central acting?

5. Indicate some of the side effects of the vagolytic action of the atropine group of drugs used for their action on the gastro-intestinal tract.

6. What do we mean by "rebound acidity" in the use of antacids in the treatment of peptic ulcer?

7. Indicate other disadvantages of some of the antacids.

8. Most vermifuges are highly toxic if absorption into the blood stream occurs. What special precautions should be taken in the administration of these drugs?

16

TREATMENT OF RESPIRATORY SYSTEM DISORDERS

The respiratory system consists of the nose, paranasal sinuses (ethmoid, sphenoid, frontal and maxillary), larynx, tracheo-bronchial tree (trachea, bronchi and their smaller divisions), and lungs. The tracheo-bronchial tree conducts the inspired air from the nose and mouth to the lungs. Although the function of the paranasal sinuses is not clear, they may serve to provide moisture to the inspired air. The larynx contains the vocal cords and together with the rest of the respiratory system is concerned with the production of sounds and words. The act of breathing brings air into intimate contact with the blood circulating through the lungs so that gaseous exchange between them may take place.

In inspiration the current of air is brought down the tracheo-bronchial tree to the lungs by a downward movement of the diaphragm; in expiration, an upward movement of the diaphragm produces an outward current, expelling the air from the lungs. The rhythmic movements of respiration are controlled in the brain by a small area designated as the respiratory center. This center is responsive to reflexes, hormones and chemical changes in the blood. Impulses from it are mediated through the phrenic nerves which run down the neck into the chest. Respiration is sometimes assisted both by movements of the ribs which enlarge the thoracic cage, and movements of the neck muscles. These accessory movements of respiration are especially prominent in states of respiratory distress.

The lining of the tracheo-bronchial tree is covered with small hair or cilia, which produce a current upward toward the mouth. This is a provision for the removal of mucus and foreign material from the tracheo-bronchial tree and lungs. The expulsion of foreign
200

material and mucus is often assisted by the cough, an abrupt and convulsive movement of the diaphragm usually excited by local irritation in the tracheo-bronchial tree. The outer surface of the lungs is covered with a glistening material, the pleura, which normally is moistened or lubricated by a small amount of pleural fluid. This makes possible the free and easy movements of the lungs against the inside of the chest cavity.

The principal function of respiration is gaseous exchange between inspired air and blood. This occurs only in the alveoli, the small air cells of the lungs. Here the blood circulating through the lungs gives up the carbon dioxide it has picked up elsewhere in the body and replaces it with oxygen which it gets from the freshly inspired air in the alveoli. If this aspect of respiratory function is to be effective both the circulation of blood through the lungs and the supply of air to the alveoli must be adequate.

Disturbances in Respiratory Function

Disturbances in respiratory function occur in infections of the paranasal sinuses, irritation and infections of the tracheo-bronchial tree, obstruction to the passage of air to the lungs, inflammation, infection, and defects in the substance of the lungs, infection and inflammation of the pleura and allergic states. In addition, there are nonpulmonary disturbances which also alter respiratory function. The common symptoms of respiratory disturbances which require treatment are cough, pain, bronchial spasm, dyspnea, orthopnea, cyanosis.

Any abnormality which reduces the amount of oxygen available (suffocation), the ability of the blood to carry oxygen (anemia), the circulation through the lungs (heart disease), or the ability of the lungs to oxygenate blood (pulmonary disease), may produce serious respiratory symptoms. Prolonged anoxia of tissues, or tissue suffocation, regardless of the cause, may produce serious and irreversible tissue damage.

Respiratory Stimulants

Respiratory stimulants are drugs which increase the rate of respiration by stimulating the respiratory center of the brain. Normally the respiratory center is sensitive to both concentration of carbon dioxide and increased acidity in the blood. As blood carbon dioxide content increases in concentration the rate of respiration increases so that a proportionately large amount may be exhaled in the expired air. There are situations however, in which the respiratory center is depressed. In such a case respiration may be exceedingly slow or even cease although the oxygen content of the blood is low and the carbon dioxide content is high. In this situation respiration must be stimulated or serious tissue damage may occur. Asphyxia, whatever its cause, is one of the most urgent emergencies in medicine. Respiration may be artificially induced in such cases, either manually or with a respirator, forcing the lungs to expel old air and take in fresh. The simpler method of treatment, however, is to use a drug to start spontaneous respiration.

Drugs which start spontaneous respiration are called respiratory stimulants and act directly on the respiratory center. Sometimes an irritant gas such as the ammonia given off by smelling salts may cause a few spontaneous gasps, but it must be recalled that a gas cannot stimulate or improve any state of asphyxia in a person who is not breathing at all, unless it is used in conjunction with artificial respiration of some kind. Carbon dioxide gas is probably the most potent respiratory stimulant but, because it is a gas, it is useful only if there is some breathing. In cases in which there is no breathing a central respiratory stimulant, such as an analeptic drug, may be injected with some effect.

Gases

Gases may be used to assist in respiratory distress. In cases in which there is no spontaneous respiration, they must be used in conjunction with some mechanical device, such as a respirator, which removes the old air from the lungs and introduces the new gas deep in the respiratory tract. In this connection it must also be mentioned that in very rapid respiration, little gas is exchanged in each breath; little, if any, of the gas in the lungs is removed and none introduced with the shallow rapid inspiration. A gas such as oxygen must be introduced efficiently if it is to accomplish anything under these circumstances. In cases when the patient is able to breathe, gas may be administered through a nasal catheter, a mask or in an enclosed tent. Although the first two are far less expensive than using a tent for administration, they are more disagreeable for the patient. An additional advantage in using a tent is seen in the summertime when the cooled tent provides a welcome kind of air-conditioning.

Oxygen

Oxygen may be given to patients who suffer from an insufficient amount of oxygen in the blood. It must be borne in mind, however, that even though oxygen so used is almost pure and about five times the concentration found in air, it can increase the oxygenation of the blood by only a small amount. While there are a large number of cases in which this small difference in the oxygen content of the blood provided by pure oxygen inhalation is a life-saving measure, there are also many instances in which little is accomplished when it is used. Oxygen is often mixed with small amounts of carbon dioxide to stimulate the respiratory center, since large amounts of pure oxygen may depress spontaneous respiration. There is a tendency, however, to expect far more from oxygen than it can give. But when it is given, it inspires confidence in many patients and their relatives that an important therapeutic measure is being provided. This is especially so when the patient is in such an impressive apparatus as a tent.

Oxygen with Helium

Oxygen with helium, given under considerable pressure, has been used in the treatment of attacks of asthma and pulmonary edema. The purpose of the abnormally high pressure is to suppress the exudation of fluid from the capillary bed into the alveoli of the lungs.

Respiratory Depressants

Respiratory depressants also act directly on the respiratory center. Such an action may occasionally be useful in cases in which the respiratory rate is so rapid as to make respiration ineffectual. It may also be effective in cases of painful respiration which tend to be very shallow as a consequence of the pain. It is to be remembered that depression of the respiratory center is a serious matter, and in most instances may be considered a toxic action. The most effective (and dangerous) respiratory depressant used is morphine, which also suppresses the cough reflex.

Mucus Suppressants

Mucus suppressants reduce the amount of mucus produced in the tracheo-bronchial tree since excessive amounts may often cause severe distress. In a patient receiving anesthesia, it may interfere with inhalation and a smooth course. It is to be remembered that mucus production by local irritant action in the bronchi and trachea is a protective mechanism and that it should be suppressed carefully and with due consideration to its cause. The common drug used for mucus suppression is atropine.

Antispasmodics

Spasm of the smooth muscle of the bronchi which causes severe respiratory distress is treated by antispasmodics. Spasm is seen most often in attacks of allergic asthma and after poisoning by irritant gases. The drugs most frequently used for bronchial dilatation are aminophylline and epinephrine. This is also discussed in the section under allergic reactions (page 206).

Cough Suppressants

Cough suppressants are used in cases in which cough causes serious distress. Since cough in general is part of a useful reflex which removes irritant material from the bronchial tree, its complete suppression may sometimes be harmful. On the other hand, too much coughing may be disabling and disturb the patient's rest; in such cases suppression may be justified. There is also the type of cough which is nonproductive and may be completely suppressed in safety but, in this case, the cough reflex does not serve any useful purpose. Sometimes the nonproductive cough is better treated by an expectorant which makes the cough a more satisfactory experience and helps to remove the irritant materials, than by a drug which suppresses the cough and prevents the removal of irritants.

Expectorants are used in instances in which the cough is nonproductive, or in which the mucus is so tenuous as to make its removal especially difficult or painful. Expectorants may increase the amount of coughing, but may make the act of coughing an easier and less painful one. On the other hand since the expectorant makes the mucus less tenuous, it often actually reduces the amount of coughing.

A nonproductive cough does not relieve the irritation which causes it and thus tends to become violent and painful and may even cause vomiting. Such paroxysms of coughing may be an exhausting experience for the patient. In such instances the therapeutic objective is to liquify the mucus of the tracheo-bronchial tree so that coughing is free, easy and productive, instead of being dry, hacking and painful. It is to be remembered that all expectorants are likely to be nauseant drugs and that there is a physiologic relationship between nausea and production of bronchial secretions. Thus patients receiving expectorants may suffer gastric upsets because of the medication.

Infections

Infections in the respiratory system are numerous and common; the following are but a few of the infections: common cold, sinusitis, pharyngitis, laryngitis, tracheitis, bronchitis, pneumonitis (pneumonias), lung abscess, pleuritis (pleurisy), tuberculosis. The treatment of the common cold, sinusitis and some of the other common infections of the upper part of the respiratory tract is still generally unsatisfactory and in much the same state as fifty years ago. Serious complications, however, are not as common now because of the antibiotics. Many of the more serious infections of the lungs have, fortunately, yielded wholly or in part to the new drugs. In recent years the problem of the treatment of bacterial and virus pneumonia has been reduced from one of the first importance to a relatively minor one. In the case of tuberculosis too, advances of importance have already been established and there are good prospects that still more important improvements are in the making. Experience with such drugs as streptomycin, para-aminosalicylic acid and isonicotinic acid hydrazide have already indicated important therapeutic uses. An account of these drugs is given in greater detail in the section on antibiotics and chemotherapeutic drugs (pages 72 to 83).

Allergic Disorders

Allergic diseases of the respiratory system, hayfever and asthma, are common and distressing conditions. Often it is possible to discover the causative allergen and to treat the condition specifically. Where the cause cannot be removed or treated, good relief may be obtained by the use of the antihistaminic drugs. In general, because of these new agents, hayfever is not the stubborn and tiresome problem it once was. In the case of asthma, unfortunately, the problem has not yielded so well to the new drugs.

Asthma

There are forms of asthma which must be differentiated from allergic asthma, for the treatment is considerably different. Cardiac asthma, as explained elsewhere (page 158) is a form of heart failure, and drugs like epinephrine, which may relieve an attack of the allergic form of asthma, may cause serious damage in the cardiac form. Cardiac asthma is treated as a problem in heart failure.

In cases of allergic asthma which do not respond to desensitization or antihistaminic drugs, epinephrine usually gives relief. This drug may be given by injection or by inhalation through a nebulizer. It is a matter of importance that the concentrated (1:100) solution used for the nebulizer should *never* be given by injection for it may produce disastrous effect due to an overdosage. Some drugs of the sympathomimetic group, ephedrine and similar drugs, may be useful substitutes for epinephrine in asthma. When this is the case, they have the additional advantage of oral administration. Unfortunately, in severe cases, the more potent and dependable epinephrine is usually necessary. All the sympathomimetic drugs may cause anxiety, nervousness and wakefulness. This may sometimes be counteracted successfully with the barbiturate drugs.

In especially serious and persistent asthmatic attacks (status asthmaticus) which have not responded to epinephrine, heroic measures are sometimes advisable. In such cases, patients may be anesthetized. In recent years, however, cortisone and ACTH have been tried and have already proved to be exceedingly useful in many such cases.

Nasal Decongestion

Because nasal congestion is one of the most common symptoms of the respiratory system nasal decongestion is a very common procedure. The usual causes of this condition are the common cold and hayfever. There is as yet no specific cure for the common cold and much treatment is directed toward the relief of the congestion in the nose so that the patient may breathe without distress. The drugs used for this symptom are usually the sympathomimetic drugs, ephedrine applied topically in solution or sometimes inhaled as a vapor. The relief which these materials afford is sometimes gratifying, but often of such short duration that repeated dosage may become the rule. Continued use of these materials by some patients may cause reaction of the nasal mucosa which eventually is more disagreeable and serious than the cold. In the case of hayfever the same drugs are used, with the same results and the same dangers.

Drugs Used in Treatment of Respiratory Disorders

Allergenic extracts	Decongestants (nasal)
Antibiotics	Expectorants
Antihistaminics	Gases
Antispasmodics	Hormones
Chemotherapeutics	Respiratory depressants
Cough suppressants	Respiratory stimulants

Study Questions

1. Review the anatomy and physiology of the respiratory tract.
2. What are the prerequisites for effective respiratory function?
3. What is the normal means by which respiration is stimulated?
4. Cough remedies usually contain what major constituents? Why?
5. What drugs are used to relieve bronchial spasm? To what general groups of drugs do these belong?
6. Many products are on the market which are used for the relief of nasal congestion. To what group of drugs do most of these belong? What is their specific action? Give examples.

17

TREATMENT OF ENDOCRINE DISORDERS

In order for the body to operate efficiently as a whole, the activity of its organs and their interrelationship is under the dual control of the nervous system and the endocrine system. The first controls activity by nervous impulses emanating from the brain and spinal cord, the latter by hormones formed in several widely distributed glands which reach the other organs and tissues through the bloodstream. The nervous and endocrine systems complement each other, and each can affect the activity of the other. In addition, the endocrine system has a profound effect on growth, development, sexual maturation, fertility and childbirth.

The endocrine system consists of several well-developed glands some of whose functions in body economy are now well defined (pituitary, thyroid, parathyroid, adrenals, ovaries and testicles, and the Islets of Langerhans of the pancreas). There are other organs whose relationship to endocrine activity is not so clearly established and is still uncertain (pineal, thymus, liver, spleen). The endocrine glands are to be distinguished from other glands of the body in that their products are absorbed directly into the bloodstream and are not conducted through ducts—hence their other name, ductless glands.

The known functions of the endocrine glands cannot be discussed here because they are too numerous and complex. The reader is referred to the brief discussions of each glandular extract listed in the Materia Medica, as well as to texts on physiology for still more detailed considerations of their functions and interrelationships. Briefly, as a group they are concerned with fertilization, intra-uterine development, birth, extra-uterine growth and development, muscular activity, intelligence, reaction to danger, reaction to infections, menstruation, ovulation, fertility, sexual drive, interest and potency, secondary sexual characteristics such as voice, hair distribution, breast development and body configuration, blood pressure, heart rate, utilization of carbohydrate, bone growth, water balance and others. Any of these may become abnormal as the result of an endocrine disturbance.

Several endocrine glands, the pituitary and adrenal glands especially, are extremely complex and produce a number of hormones, each with different functions. In general, the pituitary gland is considered to be the master gland which controls all other endocrine glands, as well as several other body functions. The interrelationship between the endocrine glands is such that in cases in which the primary disease lies in a single gland, other endocrine gland functions are likely also to be disturbed. The vital functions of the body and its development are so closely bound to the development and activity of the endocrine system that endocrine disturbances may cause the most diffuse kind of symptoms.

Endocrine Disease

Endocrine disease may be of two basic types: that of excessive production, the hyper-type, and that of insufficient function, the hypo-type. Glandular disturbances are rarely pure (of one gland alone) because underactivity of one gland may cause compensatory changes in others. It is important, therefore, to determine the basic disturbance in order to treat the disease rationally.

Endocrine disease may result from congenital malformations, infectious diseases, tumors, nutritional deficiencies and degenerative disease. The symptoms of endocrine disease are varied and diffuse: growth and developmental disturbances in the skeleton which result in dwarfs, giants, midgets, distortion of hands, feet, or face; developmental defects in sex organs and reproductive system resulting in eunuchs, sterility, impotence, frigidity, excessive sexual drive, spontaneous abortion; developmental disturbances in the body resulting in obesity, excessive thinness, effeminate body in males or masculine bodies in females, baldness, excessive hair, unusual distribution of hair, high blood pressure, headaches, excessive perspiration, unusual appetites, excessive weight loss or gain, sleepiness, dullness, excessive activity, nervousness, weakness, excessive urination; some well established disease syndromes, such a diabetes mellitus, Simmond's disease, Addison's disease, Cushing's syndrome, acromegaly, hyper- and hypothyroidism, myxedema, menopause, status thymiocolymphaticus, Graves's disease.

Treatment

Wherever possible endocrine disorders are treated by removing the cause of the disturbance. In cases of infections or tumors, this can sometimes be done with good results; the infection can be cured, or the tumor can be removed surgically and a normal state restored. This does not always happen because the infection may destroy part or all of the gland (as in the case of Addison's disease of the adrenal) or the surgical removal of the tumor may leave too little of the intact gland to serve the needs of the body.

In general, medical treatment is divided into two aspects: (1) the substitution of glandular extracts in conditions in which a hormone is deficient, and (2) attempts to depress the activity of hyperactive glands.

Endocrine Underactivity

In the first case, when glandular extracts are available, substitution therapy may be exceedingly effective. Good examples are to be found in the use of insulin in diabetes, thyroid in myxedema and the estrogenic hormones in menopause. It is to be remembered that such substitution therapy does not cure but merely provides what the body lacks; this treatment must usually be continued indefinitely. It is fortunate that there are so many glandular extracts which may be used in cases of hypoactivity of endocrine glands. It is to be borne in mind that often hormones used in therapy tend to depress the formation of the same material in the body and that after cessation of treatment the activity of the gland in question may be more depressed than previously.

Endocrine Overactivity

The problem is not so simple when glands are too active. In many instances, such as hyperactivity of the Islets of Langerhans, or parathyroid, surgical removal is the only recourse. Exceptional surgical judgment is required in deciding how much of an abnormal gland to remove. Where surgery is excessive, replacement therapy is required thereafter; where it is insufficient, more surgery is required.

Thiouracil; Iodine: One type of glandular hyperactivity, that of the thyroid gland, can be effectively treated by the use of propyl thiouracil and other thiouracil derivatives to depress thyroid activity. Another drug long of importance in thyroid disease is iodine. This drug is selectively picked up from the blood by the thyroid gland and is an essential element of the thyroid hormone, thyroxin. In general, iodine tends to regularize thyroid function, depressing activity in hyperthyroidism and stimulating it in certain types of hypothyroidism. This use is to be distinguished from that of radio-iodine (I^{131}), discussed below. Iodine is often used in conjunction with propyl thiouracil. In many instances these measures merely prepare the patient for surgery, in other cases the thiouracil seems to solve the problem without surgery.

Radiation: X-ray stands in a special position here. This modality may be used to depress glandular function but has many drawbacks in addition to the usual hazards of x-ray therapy. The chief drawback is that it is not possible to radiate the gland in question without also radiating perfectly normal tissue around it. This is especially important since most endocrine glands are in close relation to other vital structures likely to be injured by x-ray.

Of the radioactive elements recently introduced into glandular therapy, radioiodine is by far the most useful because it is the only one which is concentrated virtually exclusively in one gland, the thyroid gland. Here it produces the same effect as that of x-ray without significant radiation elsewhere. It is already established as a useful agent in the treatment of hyperthyroidism.

Synthetic Hormones: A word may be added about the synthetic hormones, a few of which are presently being used, especially in the field of estrogen therapy in the form of synthetic estrogen. There seem to be no real disadvantages in the synthetic substitutes but one general question is still unsettled. There is a possibility that the impure natural estrogens may contain certain unknown materials in addition to the hormones known to be present. It is felt by some that these unknown materials, not present in the pure synthetic form, might contribute something of importance in treatment. This is not a substantial argument against the synthetic materials since no one has been able to demonstrate superior results from the crude natural mixtures of estrogens.

There is considerable use of hormonal drugs in situations in which a clear diagnosis of insufficiency has not been made. Hormones have been used as stimulants, for weakness, for obesity, for lethargy, for lack of appetite, for excessive thinness and for a variety of uncertain indications. In many instances events may later prove that a subclinical hormonal deficiency did, in fact, exist, and if this was so, hormonal therapy will have been effective. In any event, when the indications are not clear, the use of hormones must be especially carefully followed.

Cortisone and Corticotropin (ACTH)

In many ways cortisone and corticotropin are as extraordinary and the recent discovery of these drugs is as basic and important as that of the antibiotics. The introduction of these powerful hormones marks the beginning of a fundamentally different approach to the treatment of a group of widespread serious and crippling diseases. The development of hydrocortisone which has similar actions but practical advantages has expanded the utility of this group of drugs.

Cortisone and corticotropin are still in a relatively experimental stage, certain of their applications are still unsettled, some of their long-term effects may not yet be known and many practical applications have outstripped clear understanding. Nevertheless, they have been used so widely and so much has been written about them that, even at this early stage in their development, definitive and relatively substantial statements can be made about their actions, effects, uses, limitations and dangers.

These two materials are given special consideration here, far more than for any of the other hormones, not only because of their theoretic and practical importance but also because of their newness. For only a limited amount of information is to be found about them in the textbooks on pharmacology now in print. Accordingly a relatively extensive and detailed discussion follows.

The introduction of these drugs for the treatment of arthritis in 1948 and 1949 was greeted with enthusiasm and, despite their initial scarcity, exceedingly high price, great potency and mysterious actions, their use expanded more rapidly than perhaps that of any other group of drugs in the history of medicine. This was largely so because medicaments with their particular properties were so urgently needed. The evidence was clear at the very beginning that these drugs did not cure disease, but the diseases in which they were effective in relieving symptoms were so poorly controlled by the existing measures and the need for help was so great (more people, for example, are crippled by arthritis than any other single disease) that their importance was instantly appreciated and their use expanded almost more rapidly than the drugs became available.

Cortisone was introduced for the relief of rheumatoid arthritis but, shortly after, its usefulness along with that of ACTH, in rheumatic fever and in an impressive list of other incurable diseases was discovered. Because the range of effectiveness of these drugs was not known, the agents have been tried in virtually every disease for which existing treatment is unsatisfactory and, strangely enough, in many instances dramatic relief has been obtained.

In addition to their extraordinary therapeutic effects, the response to these drugs in certain poorly understood and obscure diseases has shed new light on the nature of these diseases and has indicated a relationship between diseases which were formerly considered unrelated. The strange effects of these drugs has revolutionized our thinking about certain aspects of glandular and metabolic responses to stress, alarm and anxiety and has provided new knowledge of the scope of endocrine function.

Cortisone and ACTH are potent hormones with powerful and sometimes disturbing effects on the most fundamental metabolic functions of the animal body; they are capable of producing strange upheavels in basic physiologic responses. Their final position in physiology and medicine is not completely established but it is clear that they are hormones of the greatest importance in health as well as disease.

Cortisone is one of perhaps twenty-five steroidal materials which the cortex of the adrenal gland elaborates and then circulates throughout the body. ACTH is elaborated by the master gland, the anterior pituitary; it is the hormone which normally stimulates the adrenal cortex.

To designate these drugs as adrenal and pituitary hormones is to avoid the problem of giving them a more precise and a more descriptive name. No entirely adequate terms for them have been proposed; in this book we have chosen to call them mesenchymal hormones, a term not likely to be found in other texts. At this stage in our knowledge this descriptive term seems useful because it indicates the nature of their most important therapeutic actions, namely that on the mesenchymal tissues. We know, of course, that they have other important spheres of influence in body function, but many of these comprise undesirable rather than therapeutic effects.

Cortisone (compound E, cortone, cortogen) is a crystalline steroidal hormone extracted from the cortex of the adrenal gland (commercially from cattle and now also synthesized from bile). ACTH (officially called corticotropin, scientifically called the adrenocorticotropic hormone, commercially called acthar) is a purified hormone extracted from the anterior pituitary gland of cattle. These hormones are normally excreted in minute amounts by the same gland in man and play a fundamental role in health as well as in disease, especially in the reaction of the body to disease and the development of symptoms. ACTH stimulates the cortex of the adrenal gland to produce cortisone as well as other related steroidal materials. ACTH also stimulates other unrelated endocrine functions. Our present interest in ACTH lies in the fact that it increases the production of cortisone by the adrenal cortex and that its major therapeutic actions derive largely from this cortisone. As might be expected, its therapeutic effects are much the same as that of cortisone.

Effects on Tissues

The therapeutic effect of cortisone and ACTH on tissues seems largely restricted to mesenchymal or connective tissues. It prevents or restrains the reactions to cellular insults (injuries) such as that due to infection, trauma, chemicals, heat, allergy, etc. The drugs do not attack the cause, they do not stimulate the resistance of the body against injury, they do not help in cure or in the repair of injury, they merely restrain reactions to injury. Given in exceedingly large doses these drugs may completely suppress all inflammatory reactions regardless of cause.

The therapeutic value of this strange effect lies in the fact that in many diseases, the body's defense against insult is excessive, the response is not a well balanced one and some overreactions not only causes severe symptoms but may also leave permanent injuries to organs as a result of the defense reaction itself. It is well to emphasize that the permanent scarring of organs in some diseases, seen after the disease is cured, is not due directly to the pathologic effects of the disease-producing agent but to a residual effect of the body's defenses against the disease. By restraining such exuberant responses to insult, cortisone and ACTH may prevent permanent organ damage and in other cases they may suppress or relieve severe symptoms which are secondary to excessive inflammation.

Therapeutic Effects

This restraining action of cortisone and ACTH is especially valuable, therefore, in diseases which are characterized by excessive inflammatory reactions and in diseases in which the symptoms and the permanent effects are largely the result of the reactions to disease rather than the result of the etiologic agent itself. It is well to remember that these drugs do not cure, on the contrary, they restrain what we often designate as defense mechanisms.

It is important to bear in mind also, that the doses of cortisone and ACTH used therapeutically far exceed the amounts of these same materials which may normally be excreted by the adrenal cortex and the pituitary gland. These drugs are not used for adrenal or pituitary insufficiency; this is not replacement therapy in the sense that insulin in diabetes, thyroid in myxedema and estrogens in menopause are used to replace a hormone in a condition in which the body produces insufficient amounts in which case an amount is given which brings the amount in the body up to normal levels. The mesenchymal hormones are used in unusually large and what might be considered abnormal doses in the endeavor to depress a normal reaction of the body to attack the inflammatory reaction. It is to be expected, therefore, that such abnormal doses can also produce therapeutically undesirable effects as well.

Rheumatoid Arthritis

In this condition the permanent injury and crippling is due to inflammatory reaction in joints with exudation, fibrosis and anky-losis of joints as the final event. This disease has been resistant to all types of treatment and, in general, even relief is difficult to obtain. Gold therapy, which was the most effective treatment before the introduction of cortisone, did not relieve all patients, in many the relief was short-lived and, in addition, the drug was dangerous, often followed by serious reactions, could be used only for limited periods and with limited dosage, and required great skill and ex-perience for its proper administration. It was often a drug of last resort.

Virtually all patients with rheumatoid arthritis respond dramat-ically to cortisone and ACTH. The fever subsides, the sedimentation rate falls, and very soon stiff joints can move without pain. The patients feel better, stronger, take more interest in life, food, sex. With such rapid improvement the patient regains assurance about his outlook. Unfortunately, in most cases, despite the promptness and the extent of improvement, as soon as medication is discon-tinued symptoms are likely to return.

Rheumatic Fever

Rheumatic fever frequently causes serious heart disease in children; it has been called Children's Public Enemy Number One. In this disease the damage to the heart valves is the result of excessive inflammatory reaction during the acute phase of the dis-ease, which, after the disease subsides, does not disappear com-pletely but leaves a scar on the valve. Cortisone and ACTH can suppress the inflammatory reaction, reduce the swelling and the pain in the joints, and make the patient more comfortable and less toxic than any other therapeutic agent. After the drug is given the fever subsides, the sedimentation rate falls, the electrocardiogram returns to normal and the patient who was very ill feels remarkably well and happy.

In some cases in which the restraining influences of these drugs were applied early in the course of the disease and before perma-nent damage to the heart valves occurred, and in which therapy was continued throughout the inflammatory stage of the disease, permanent or, at least, serious cardiac damage had been averted. Some such cases have not even developed transient murmurs during the acute stage. Thus, while the disease is not cured by these drugs, the patient may nontheless be served just as well as if a specific cure were available, for the only serious complication of the disease may be prevented.

Collagen Diseases

Cortisone and ACTH are used in a group of obscure diseases which are now thought to be related to rheumatoid arthritis and rheumatic fever, the so-called collagen diseases. These are fundamentally diseases of the connective tissues; each disease being a somewhat different manifestation of collagen disease. Many of them are rare, incurable and usually fatal. The causes are unknown. They include periarteritis nodosa, lupus erythematosis, scleroderma and dermatomyositis. The drugs do not cure but, as in the case of arthritis, they offer the only means of staying the course of the disease and relieving symptoms.

Eye

The eye is one of the most delicate as well as one of the most precious organs. Inflammations of the eye, even those due to inconsequential infections or irritants may induce severe reactions of the cornea and other ocular structures and may result in partial or complete blindness. In such cases cortisone and ACTH may save sight by restraining these inflammatory reactions. Here again, the drugs do not cure, they merely restrain reactions to injury, but in doing so they perform a vital function. The effect is now used in many ocular diseases as well as in mechanical and chemical injuries and, in general, in emergencies of the eye.

Allergy

In much the same way cortisone and ACTH restrain the allergic response to allergens; sometimes very dramatically in situations in which the patient's life is endangered by the extent of the allergic reaction and in which no other agents offer relief. Cortisone and ACTH are now commonly used in preference to all other agents in instances of severe status asthmaticus, drug reactions, skin eruptions and urticaria.

Miscellaneous Conditions

Cortisone and ACTH are also used in a variety of unrelated diseases in which they afford some relief. They are often used in diseases of the adrenal gland such as Addison's disease, in the preoperative stages of Cushing's disease and in the Waterhouse-Friderichsen syndrome. They are also sometimes used in malignant diseases, with especially useful effects in the leukemias.

Untoward Effects

The untoward effects which may follow their use may be grave, but with our present understanding, with proper regulation of dosage and with consideration for the indications, unwarranted and serious complications may be avoided. It is well to bear in mind that these drugs are deliberately used in unphysiologic doses to produce what, under normal circumstances, would be considered unphysiologic effects; that serious results might follow is, therefore, not surprising. It is fortunate indeed that in most cases untoward effects disappear soon after the drugs are discontinued.

Adrenal Gland

Cortisone (but not ACTH) depresses the activity of the adrenal cortex and, as a consequence, the long continued use of cortisone may induce profound and persistent depression of the gland. In such a case, when the cortisone is discontinued, immediately thereafter there may be a period of severe adrenal insufficiency. ACTH which, in effect, works by stimulating the adrenal cortex does not produce this effect. It has recently been recommended that, when cortisone is used for a protracted period, the treatment be interrupted by short courses of ACTH to stimulate the activity of the adrenal cortex and to prevent sustained depression of the gland which may be produced when the cortisone is used without such an interruption.

Electrolyte Disturbances

Both cortisone and ACTH cause retention of sodium and water.

In cases in which this effect is substantial or in patients especially sensitive to such an effect, for example those with serious heart disease, it may precipitate symptoms of heart failure with edema and even ascites. In part, this may be controlled by the limitation of salt in the diet and the use of diuretics. The drugs may interfere with the control of heart failure in patients with heart disease who are given the cortisone or ACTH for some other condition.

Cortisone and ACTH also increase the rate of potassium and chloride excretion, an effect which may result in alkalosis with symptoms of weakness, low blood pressure, arrhythmias and electrocardiographic disturbances.

Blood Pressure

Cortisone and ACTH may stimulate a moderate increase in blood pressure. This possibility may be a matter of importance only in patients who have high blood pressure. In such patients the effect on the blood pressure should be carefully followed.

Carbohydrate Metabolism

Cortisone and ACTH decrease the responsiveness to insulin and elevate blood sugar levels. In normal patients this may result in a transient glycosuria, while in diabetic patients it may interfere with the established control of the diabetes. This disturbance may be prevented by an appropriate increase in insulin dosage during cortisone or ACTH therapy. The effect on carbohydrate metabolism disappears promptly after withdrawing the drug. It is well to remember this in the case of the diabetic whose insulin dosage has been raised, for if the insulin is not appropriately decreased when the cortisone or ACTH are discontinued, the patient may suffer an insulin reaction.

Protein Metabolism

Large doses of cortisone and ACTH tend to increase the destruction of protein in the body and to produce a negative nitrogen balance despite the ingestion of large amounts of protein.

Healing of Wounds

By restraining the activity of mesenchymal tissue reaction to injury, cortisone and ACTH also retard the healing of wounds which, of course, represents a form of tissue insult; these drugs may delay healing of wounds whether caused by injury, surgery or disease. This is a strange reversal of the same mechanism which is used to prevent the damaging effects of other diseases. The restraint to wound healing may be a serious matter in some cases and necessitate the cessation of the drugs until after the wounds have healed.

Skin

In many instances these drugs are followed by the appearance of acne. The condition usually disappears promptly after the drugs are discontinued.

Sexual Function

Sexual physiology is disturbed by cortisone and ACTH. These drugs increase the production of the androgenic hormones, an effect which usually increases sexual interest and drive and which, in the female, may also induce a degree of masculinization, excessive hair, acne, deepened voice and disturbances in menstruation. All return to their former state when the drug is discontinued.

Psychic Effects

It has already been indicated that after receiving cortisone and ACTH patients feel much better and complain less. This seems to be due only in part to the relief of symptoms and to the indication to the patient that at last something positive is being done about a devastating and apparently hopeless condition. There also seems to be a sense of well-being, which appears promptly after the drug is given and before there is appreciable symptomatic relief, which is the result of direct psychic action of the drugs. It is this frame of mind which will so often make the patient insist on the continuation of the drug regardless of the medical indications to stop it.

The sense of well-being may progress to a state of marked elation or even euphoria; in some cases to a state of mania. Sleep may be disturbed and extraordinary swings of mood may develop.

Rarely is there depression. Psychic effects tend to subside promptly. Sometimes patients lean so heavily on the drugs, as to simulate addiction.

Blood Clotting

Large doses of cortisone and ACTH may increase the prothrombin time of blood, an affect which may interfere with blood clotting.

Masking of Infections

Because these drugs suppress reactions of the body to infections there is the possibility that during the course of prolonged treatment of a chronic disease with cortisone or ACTH an unrelated infection may develop without producing a symptom or other warning signal of its presence. The importance of this possibility lies not only in the effects of an unrecognized and untreated infection in the patient but also that, ignorant of the infection, the patient may spread it to others. Chief among such dangerous possibilities is pulmonary tuberculosis. It is good precaution, therefore, for patients who receive these drugs regularly to have a chest x-ray every six months.

Contraindications

Special difficulties may be encountered when cortisone and ACTH are used in patients who have the following conditions: (1) heart disease, especially with congestive failure; (2) hypertension; (3) renal insufficiency (not including nephrosis); (4) diabetes; (5) peptic ulcer; (6) psychic instability; (7) wounds, especially surgical incisions. None are, however, absolute contraindications, for with careful supervision cortisone and ACTH may be used in these conditions without serious trouble.

The Agent of Choice

In general, the difference in the therapeutic indications for these two agents are minute and often unclear or not well established. Much depends on the precise state of the disease as well as on the experience of the physician. Cortisone presents advantages in oral administration which may be effective, usually after a period of parenteral administration. Its effects are, in general, not likely to be as diffuse as ACTH because it does not involve as many other glandular functions. Its chief disadvantage lies in the depression of the adrenal gland.

ACTH must be injected. It does not depress the adrenal gland but, on the other hand, the adrenal gland must be responsive or ACTH cannot stimulate the production of cortisone. ACTH influences the activity of other glands, a fact which is sometimes a therapeutic advantage, sometimes a disadvantage.

Hydrocortisone is another adrenal steroid hormone, closely allied to cortisone but not identical or derived from it. It has just become commercially available. It has the advantage of local effectiveness without systemic actions. It is used for its effects on joints by direct injection into joint cavities.

Drugs Used in Treatment of Endocrine Disorders

Androgens

Antithyroids

Adrenals

Estrogens (natural)

Estrogens (synthetic)

Hormones

Insulins

Parathormones

Pituitaries (anterior lobe)

Pituitaries (posterior lobe)

Placentals

Study Questions

1. What are the various endocrine glands? Tabulate these by name and indicate their hormones with specific actions, uses, administration and toxic actions.

2. What is cortisone? What are some of its effects, uses and toxic symptoms? What is its relationship to corticotropin (ACTH)?

3. In the presence of hypofunction of many of the endocrine glands, medical treatment requires substitution therapy. Give examples.

4. What is the action of the iodine and the thiouracil drugs in the treatment of thyrotoxicosis? Indicate their effects.

5. What is the principle of action and effectiveness of radioactive iodine?

TREATMENT OF
REPRODUCTIVE SYSTEM DISORDERS

The reproductive systems of the two sexes differ; in the male it is comprised of the testicles (or gonads), the seminal vesicles, the prostate gland and the penis; in the female it consists of the ovaries (or gonads), the fallopian tubes, the uterus and the vagina. The reproductive system is largely under the control of the endocrine glands of the body, especially the hormones produced by the pituitary gland. The reproductive function of the system combines a mechanism for sexual interest, potency and fertility, and a mechanism for the fertilization of the egg with the sperm, the harboring of the fertilized egg until it is ready for birth and the entire birth process. The gonads of each sex, in addition to providing the seed for fertilization, are also endocrine glands which tend to maintain the secondary physical sexual characteristics which externally distinguish the two sexes: the distribution of hair, the voice, the configuration of the hips, the texture of the skin, the development of functional breasts. When the gonads cease to function, the secondary sexual characteristics tend to change, and the individual so afflicted tends somewhat toward a neutral state.

Dysfunction in the reproductive systems may be due to congenital defects or deficiencies in the gonads or other parts of the reproductive system, and disorders in other endocrine glands which exert some control over reproductive function. For example, disease of the pituitary, adrenal or thyroid glands may cause disturbances in the reproductive system. Infections play an important role in disturbances in this system. Eventually, age takes its toll in all people as the gonads lose their function and the symptoms which result from their deficiency in hormone production are known as climacteric or the male and female menopause.

Endocrine Disorders

Endocrine disorders which affect the reproductive system usually depress sexual activity, although there are cases in which some aspects of the mechanism are stimulated. Castration (loss of testicular or ovarian function), whether congenital or due to surgery or disease, causes changes in secondary sexual characteristics toward those of the opposite sex. One may lose sexual interest and vigor, sterility always sets in and the female ceases to menstruate. In addition, diffuse symptoms such as hot flushes, vague pains and aches, headaches, weakness and alterations in the distribution of hair and the configuration of the body may also appear.

The most logical and effective treatment of an endocrine deficiency is by replacement with the deficient hormone. This requires an accurate diagnosis. In some cases it may be thyroid or pituitary hormone which is required, but most frequently the sex hormone itself is needed. None of these hormones, however, restores fertility in patients with nonfunctioning or absent gonads, for they do not provide the necessary seed. In many cases of menopausal syndrome, the therapy can be guided by tests. The simplest and commonest of these tests now is the vaginal smear.

The estrogenic (female sex) hormones may be either natural or synthetic. The natural hormones are usually obtained from the urine of pregnant humans or animals. The synthetic hormones are usually satisfactory substitutes which have the advantage of being cheaper. An argument concerning their relative merits is given elsewhere (page 211).

As the male grows older there is a tendency for the prostate gland to enlarge. This interferes with urinary function and is usually exceedingly disturbing to the patient. The enlargement may be controlled to some extent by estrogenic therapy. Large doses are necessary and surgery often provides a simpler answer to the problem.

Androgenic (male sex) hormones may be used in the treatment of the male with menopausal symptoms and those with some loss of sexual vigor. The latter is not frequently to be recommended for it tends further to depress normal gonadal function. The androgens may also be used in the female to control excessive menstrual bleeding.

It should also be mentioned that both estrogenic and androgenic hormones may be used in the treatment of cancer of the breast and estrogenic hormone for cancer of the prostate. This is discussed in more detail in another section (page 251).

Sterility

Sterility in patients with apparently normal gonads may be caused by mechanical defects in other parts of the reproductive system or other endocrine deficiencies. Where surgical correction is not possible, the outlook for successful therapy with hormones alone is not usually good. Stimulant therapy sometimes helps in cases in which the basic defect can be identified, but unfortunately it is not often possible to establish the cause of sterility. Often sterility is relative, and after a long period of infertility, pregnancy occurs.

Abortion

Abortion is a special problem in many females who are fertile and become pregnant easily but, for some reason or other, cannot carry through the entire period of gestation. In some cases the difficulty is a mechanical one, such as a tumor of the uterus, but it is usually due to an endocrine disturbance. In this situation estrogens, other sex hormones, and pituitary hormones may be useful in the prevention of spontaneous abortion.

On the other hand, it may be stated categorically, that the use of drugs in the attempt to terminate pregnancies illegally in its later stages is futile and fraught with grave danger.

Childbirth

During the final stages of childbirth the activity of the uterus, if it is fatigued may be assisted by drugs. Pituitary extracts may stimulate labor pains and increase the force of the contractions of the uterus. After delivery of the child and placenta, ergot or extracts of ergot are usually used to reduce the bleeding; the ergot causes the uterus to clamp down on the site of the attachment of the placenta to the uterus. Ergot should never be administered before the expulsion of the placenta.

Contraception

In instances in which religious beliefs and moral convictions permit, medical indications for the use of contraceptives will be considered by the physician. He is the only person qualified to determine the presumed influence of a full-term pregnancy on the course of the disease a pregnant patient has. The effective use of contraceptives requires training, cooperation and intelligence; failure is common when these are not present, and injury is also possible. Contraceptives must not be so strong as to cause vaginal irritation; serious accidents have occurred from the use of ill-advised and potent solutions for this purpose. For example, there are many instances of serious and even fatal poisoning from the use of mercuric chloride solutions as a contraceptive douche.

Vaginal Irrigation

Vaginal irrigations are often used by women who are under the misapprehension that this is always a hygienic measure. It is to be remembered that the vagina is provided by nature with fluids and antiseptic materials of its own which maintain cleanliness and health of the vaginal mucosa. There is rarely a normal need to irrigate the vagina, and usually more harm than good comes from it. Vaginal irrigations should be used only when there are specific indications for it and are prescribed by the doctor. They should always be of the mildest materials.

Infections in the Reproductive System

Infections may develop in the reproductive system. Venereal infections may be briefly considered here. Almost invariably, venereal infections are acquired during sexual intercourse, rarely accidentally. Most of the early manifestations of venereal infections are in the external genitalia, but later, extensions and complications may involve deeper structures of the reproductive system and may extend to other organs as well. In recent years the treatment of all venereal diseases has improved dramatically and the infections which were difficult and unsatisfactory to treat, syphilis, gonorrhea, lymphogranuloma, now respond well to our new drugs and results are far more satisfactory. It seems that it should now be possible to eradicate venereal disease.

Other infections of the reproductive system are relatively rare and are treated in the standard way with chemotherapeutic and antibiotic drugs. The most serious of these illnesses, puerperal sepsis, once constituted the most frightening prospect in bearing a child; today it is a disease relatively easily treated by both chemotherapeutic and antibiotic agents.

Dysmennorhea

Dysmennorhea is so common today that it invalids a large part of our female population for a few days each month. Why this condition should apparently be on the increase is conjectural. In a few cases a defect of the reproductive system may be found which can be corrected, in some cases the condition disappears after the patient bears her first child, but in most cases no cause and, for that matter, no remedy can be found. In the latter cases, the common analgesics, such as the salicylates sometimes help. In many cases, however, these are too modest in their action and more potent analgesia is sought. This sometimes presents a grave danger of habituation by the regularly recurring use of such drugs as codeine or alcohol.

In some cases hormones, estrogenic, androgenic and ovarian may be helpful. Viburnum, once the most popular remedy for dysmenorrhea has fallen into disrepute, largely because of its ineffectiveness.

Drugs Used in Treatment of Reproductive System Disorders

Androgens	Estrogens
Antibiotics	Luteal hormones
Chemotherapeutics	Oxytocics
Ecbolics, *see* Oxytocics	Uterine sedatives

Study Questions

1. Indicate actions and uses of the male and female sex hormones.

2. What is the value and the purpose of the use of pituitary extracts and ergot preparations pre- and postnatally?

3. Why may frequent vaginal irrigations with antiseptic and other solutions, be contraindicated?

19

TREATMENT OF
URINARY SYSTEM DISORDERS

The urinary system consists of the two kidneys in which the urine is formed, the ureters which are thin tubes which conduct the urine from the kidneys to the urinary bladder, the urinary bladder in which the urine is temporarily stored and the urethra through which urine flows during urination. Because of the intimate association with the reproductive system there are some sex differences. In the male, the urethra leads through the prostate gland and penis and is relatively longer and thinner than the urethra of the female which leads directly from the bladder. In addition, the prostate gland lies in such a position that it may cause obstruction to the flow of urine through the urethra and prevent the complete emptying of the bladder; the female has no prostate gland or practical counterpart.

The kidney is a complex organ which purifies blood by removing from it the soluble wastes and water which form the urine. The rate of urine formation depends on (1) the circulation through the kidney; (2) the condition of the glomerulae of the kidney, the microscopic organs which actually filter the blood; and (3) the condition of the tubules of the kidney through which filtered water is returned to the bloodstream, thus concentrating the urine. In this way water is conserved and urination is reduced; the amount of fluid one would have to drink to provide the water necessary to make unconcentrated urine is therefore decreased.

Disturbances in Urination and Urine Formation

The frequency of urination or voiding is to be distinguished from the amount of urine formed. This depends on (1) the amount of urine formed; (2) the distention of the bladder; (3) the completeness of emptying of the bladder during voiding, for clearly if urine is left in the bladder it will fill up more quickly; (4) the chemical nature of the urine, for if it is irritant it may stimulate the desire for urination even though the bladder is empty, and (5) the presence of infection, which may also stimulate the desire to urinate.

Disturbances in urine formation and in urination are the most prominent symptoms of urinary system disorders. These may include frequency, insufficiency or complete absence of urination, painful or burning urination, difficulty in starting or stopping urination, difficulty with dribbling after urination, edema, increase of wastes in the bloodstream (uremia), coma, death. These may result from congenital or mechanical defects, irritations, inflammations or infections in any part of the tract. In addition, urinary function may be upset by diseases of other organs, the most common of these being heart disease and high blood pressure in which the circulatory inefficiency influences the rate of urine formation.

Disturbances in urination, if due to mechanical defects of one type or another, usually respond best to surgical treatment. When due to irritation, inflammation or infection, there are effective medical remedies. It has to be recalled that, until recently, infections of the urinary tract were exceedingly common and poorly treated. With the introduction of the sulfa drugs and the antibiotics, many of the common infections of the urinary tract were well treated for the first time.

Diseases of the Kidney

Disease of the kidneys may be due to (1) congenital defects, (2) stones, (3) infections, (4) heart disease, (5) vascular disease, (6) degenerative disease, (7) poisoning, (8) unknown causes. Antibiotics may sometimes be effective in the case of infections. Surgery may be used in cases of congenital or mechanical defects and stones, as well as in some cases of infections. Disturbances due to heart disease respond well if the heart function can be improved or if diuretics are used.

Nephritis

Outstanding as a therapeutic problem is nephritis, an inflammatory disease of the kidneys, of which there are two important general forms. The acute form is usually seen in early life; the chronic form is seen in young adults and older people with vascular disease such as hypertension or arteriosclerosis. Neither of these two serious diseases are responsive to specific therapy. The cause of acute nephritis is not established, and while it frequently improves spontaneously, its treatment is unsatisfactory. It often complicates pregnancy, and in such cases there may be great improvement after the child is born, but treatment per se, is not particularly helpful. Specific treatment is also unsatisfactory in the vascular diseases of the kidney and disease may continue to progress despite therapy. In all these forms of nephritis the most effective therapy available is symptomatic. Many poisons, taken deliberately or accidentally, may injure the kidneys. For some types of poisoning we have effective remedies, for others none. It usually takes a specialist to apply the best treatment.

Pain in Urinary Disturbances

Pain is a relatively common symptom in urinary disturbances and may be due to stone, inflammation or infection anywhere in the urinary tract. Pain due to stone may be of the severest the human being may have to suffer in any disease. The relief of such pain usually requires the application of the strongest agents.

Pain in urination due to infection, irritations, or inflammation in the urinary tract is often easier to relieve. The infection can be treated, the irritation or inflammation can be handled by diluting the urine through the drinking of large amounts of water, and by the use of alkali to reduce the acidity of the urine.

Diuretics

Drugs which increase the rate of urine formation by the kidneys are called diuretics. They are most frequently and effectively used in heart disease in cases of heart failure in which the rate of urine formation is depressed (page 167). They may also be used in other illnesses when it is necessary to increase the rate of urine formation. Many of the diuretics, however, will not work in instances in which no urine at all is being formed; if these drugs are to act the kidneys must be able to form urine. They are least effectual, therefore, in extensive kidney disease, whereas they provide their greatest benefits in urinary disturbances which are not due to kidney disease (i.e., heart disease). They are rarely useful in cases of poisoning, either to initiate urination or to increase the rate of excretion of poisons.

In connection with the action of the diuretics it is important to remember that the element, sodium, found in table salt and many alkaline medications and foods, tends to bind water and produce edema. In some renal diseases as well as in heart disease, therefore, effective diuretic treatment includes the restriction of salt in the diet and hastening its elimination.

Depending on the basic disease, the rate of urine formation can be accelerated by (1) correcting circulatory disturbances, (2) increasing the rate of salt elimination, (3) decreasing the rate of salt storage, (4) increasing the rate of blood filtration in the kidney glomerulae, (5) decreasing the rate at which the kidney tubules absorb the water filtered out of the bloodstream, (6) increasing the dilution of blood. The drugs selected to induce diuresis will depend on which one of these mechanisms is desired. Because the practical importance of diuretics is greater in heart disease than in others these drugs are considered in detail in that section.

Antidiuretics

Antidiuretics are drugs which decrease the rate of urine formation. Such an action is rarely needed aside from one disease, diabetes inspidus, in which there is a pathologic thirst and excessive amounts of urine are formed. While the taking of large amounts of salt will diminish the rate of urine formation it is not practical in this disease. Here a highly specific action may be obtained from the use of extract of the posterior pituitary gland or pitressin. Patients with diabetes inspidus who are virtually helpless because of almost continuous drinking and urination may be returned to a state of normal urine formation by the daily application of these glandular extracts. It is of practical importance that the pituitary extract may be applied intranasally as well as intramuscularly.

Urinary Antiseptics

Urinary antiseptics have long been used because infections of the lower part of the urinary system are exceedingly common. These agents have very limited value and for this reason, until the recent chemotherapeutic drugs and antibiotics were introduced, urinary tract infections tended to become chronic problems for patient and doctor. Often these infections are complications of defects which must be corrected surgically if a permanent cure is to be obtained. These occur in elderly males with enlarged prostate glands, in cases of stones, kinks, pockets, bends in the kidney pelvis, the ureters or bladder. Where infections are not complicated by mechanical defects, many of the common infections are relatively rapidly eliminated by the use of the sulfonamide drugs or the properly selected antibiotic. Formerly it was common to pass sounds through the urethra and to inject antiseptics directly into the bladder through a catheter. Today because of the great effectiveness of our drugs, such measures are relatively rarely practiced. It is interesting to note that at the present time, the antibiotics and chemotherapeutic agents are effective in most of the common infections of the urinary tract, and that our serious problems in treatment are with infections which formerly were very rare but have recently become more common as a result of the use of these same effective antibacterial agents.

Alkalinization and Acidification

Acidity, as has been mentioned, may stimulate the desire to urinate even when little urine is present. Such chemical irritation may be relieved by the use of common alkali such as sodium bicarbonate. In addition, alterations in urinary acidity may be essential to therapy. For example, when sulfa drugs are used, alkaline urine prevents kidney complications, when mandelic acid or methenamine are used as urinary antiseptics, acid urine is required. For acidification, acid-forming salts such as ammonium chloride, or even acids, such as hydrochloric or phosphoric acid may be used. For the alkalinization of urine, sodium bicarbonate may be used, although in cases with heart disease other alkalis not containing sodium are preferable. Potassium bicarbonate which may be used for this purpose should be handled with caution since the accumulation of the potassium ion may cause serious toxic effects, and is especially dangerous in the cardiac patient on a salt-free diet.

Stones

Stones in the urinary tract usually cause exquisite pain when they begin to move down the tract; in addition they are often the site of infection and may eventually cause chronic kidney disease through obstruction to the flow of urine and the infection. Most stones, if left to their own devices, will eventually pass spontaneously out of the urinary tract. In cases in which this does not occur the simplest and most direct way of treating the stone is to remove it surgically. Attempts may be made, however, to dissolve the stone chemically. When the nature of the stone is determined, the acidity or alkalinity of the urine may be shifted according to the solubility of the particular type of stone. Dietary measures also help in certain cases. In addition, there is evidence that the use of aluminum hydroxide gels by mouth may, by interfering with specific absorptions, prevent the development of certain types of renal stones. These measures may also be used to prevent the recurrence of stones in patients who exhibit a tendency to develop them.

Evidence has recently been adduced that hyaluronidase is excreted in the urine and that it may tend to prevent the agglutination of particles in the urine which eventually form renal stones, and that the drug may be injected subcutaneously in patients who tend to form stones for this purpose.

Drugs Used in Treatment of Urinary System Disorders

Acidifiers (urinary)	Antispasmodics
Alkalizers (urinary)	Chemotherapeutics
Antibiotics	Diuretics
Antiseptics (urinary)	

Study Questions

1. Review the anatomy and physiology of the genito-urinary tract in the male and female.

2. Upon what factors does frequency of urination depend?

3. What role does the nurse play in the treatment and prevention of urinary tract infections?

4. What are the indications and contraindications for the use of diuretics in the presence of renal disease?

5. What is the principle of action of urinary antiseptics? By what means are some of their toxic effects counteracted?

6. There are certain drugs which may be used to prevent and to treat conditions of stone formation in the urinary tract. Give examples. What is the principle of their actions?

20

TREATMENT OF
MUSCULO-SKELETAL DISORDERS

Movement of the body or any of its external parts is made possible by what may be called the musculo-skeletal system. This consists of the bony skeleton which holds the body together and provides a framework for support, and joints which permit the various kinds of movement. The extensive and powerful movements of the arms and legs, the skilled and intricate movements of the fingers, the expressive movements of the face and jaw, the limited twisting movements in the spinal column are all activities of the musculo-skeletal system. The power for these movements is provided by actively contracting muscles. Strong tendons and ligaments hold the bones together and attach the muscles to the bones. Finally, the control of these movements is provided by the nervous system, the brain which determines the nature of the voluntary as well as the involuntary movements, the nerves which carry the impulses from the brain to the muscles it directs, and the reflex arc which provides a constant tone or tension to the muscles and keeps them from being flabby when not actively and forcefully contracting. The proper integration of these makes possible smooth, coordinated, powerful, skilled and purposeful movements. A disturbance in any of these may cause muscular movements to be painful, involuntary, weak, jerky, gross, uncoordinated or purposeless.

The skeleton consists of the bones and the joints on which they move. Normally, the bones are well calcified and strong enough for normal strains and stresses, and the surfaces of the joints glisten with a smooth coating of cartilage. This surface is lubricated with small amounts of fluid and the joint is enclosed in a ligamentous capsule or envelope which holds the two articulating surfaces together. Many joints have small or larger finger-like outpocketings called bursa which communicate with the joint cavity and serve no known useful purpose.

Any or all of these structures may be affected by disease. Dietary deficiencies are frequent offenders in children, rickets (vitamin D) and scurvy (vitamin C) especially. These nutritional defects are corrected by proper diet and a sufficient amount of the needed vitamins. Disease of the parathyroid gland may affect the calcification and strength of the bones. The excessive production of the hormone of the parathyroid gland is usually corrected surgically. Bone tumors may be treated by surgery or radiation. Infections of the bone may respond to antibiotics, but surgery is also frequently required.

Pain

Pain in the musculo-skeletal system may be either diffuse or local, but it is exceedingly common. It may be present in virtually any bone, joint, or muscle. Many instances may never be serious enough to be brought to a doctor's attention and are usually treated by the patient himself with heat or some common remedy like aspirin. Thus, many of the vague pains or aches are never diagnosed. Many of these symptoms which are brought to a doctor's attention are so indefinite that they are exceedingly difficult to diagnose. In most instances, proper diagnosis is not of great practical importance for the pains respond to simple treatment and disappear permanently. In other cases, however, muscle pains and joint pains are not easily relieved by the common remedies and sometimes are related to serious disease. Such pain and aches do not respond to treatment until the proper diagnosis is made and treatment is determined on the basis of diagnosis. In many cases local physical measures involving heat will relieve the pain. Other cases will not respond until specific therapy is applied.

Arthritis

Arthritis is a disease of bones, more especially of the joints in which movement may become exquisitely painful or even impossible. The cause may be an infection, such as gonorrhea, or an acute pyogenic infection, but most frequently the cause is unknown. Arthritis may be classified as a mesenchymal disease, one of the connective tissues, bones, ligaments, muscles and so forth. This has practical bearing on its tendency to respond to cortisone and corticotropin (ACTH).

Over the years, many different remedies have been tried in arthritis; the large list attests to the number that have been useless and discarded. In many early and simple cases good relief may be obtained with simple remedies like aspirin. Local applications of heat and counter-irritants have long been used and are sometimes helpful. More recently large doses of vitamin D have been recommended although its results are questionable. Until the introduction of cortisone and corticotropin the gold salts had been the most effective remedy for arthritis. Gold helped a large number of patients with arthritis, especially the rheumatoid form, but the use of gold is attended by substantial danger from toxic reactions and it should be administered only by those with considerable experience.

The most recent contributions to the treatment of arthritis are cortisone and corticotropin (ACTH). These powerful hormones exert a profound influence on all mesenchymal disease, relieving some painful arthritic states promptly. It is unfortunate indeed, that in most instances symptoms return with discouraging promptness once therapy is stopped. In addition, these potent hormones may have serious toxic effects, for which the patient must be constantly watched. It is to be hoped that new derivatives of these drugs will soon be developed which are less dangerous, less expensive and have longer-lasting effects.

Gout

Gout, already discussed on page 150, is a metabolic disorder which frequently involves the skeletal system. Instead of excreting uric acid crystals the body deposits them around the joints. The cause of gout is not known and is apparently not directly related to the amount of food which produces uric acid which is ingested. Symptoms will appear regardless of diet in patients with a gouty tendency. The deposition of crystals in joints, usually the smaller joints of the feet or hands, make movement exquisitely painful and eventually leads to bone destruction. Many drugs may be used to relieve the pain but none are known which cure the disorder. Some of the drugs may influence the rate of uric acid excretion, but this, too, is not now thought to be important. The more effective remedies for the relief of pain in gout today are colchcine and cinchophen. Cortisone is also used.

Myalgias

Myalgias are common conditions in which there is pain and often spasm in skeletal muscle groups. Sometimes the pain can be devastating. Often no cause can be found and no other disease discovered. The stiff neck (torticollis) is a common example. There are many forms of treatment, all of which sometimes help and all of which sometimes fail. These are applications of heat, massage, salicylates, injections with procaine and spray with ethyl chloride.

Neuromuscular Disorders

Neuromuscular disorders comprise a group of mysterious, disabling diseases which are all too often incurable. The difficulty in muscular function in these disorders is in some way closely bound with a difficulty in the communication between muscle and nerve. Both primary weakness in the substance of the muscle itself and primary disease of the central nervous system occur. However, in many cases neither seems to play a part. Both organ systems seem to be normal, yet the two do not work together efficiently. These diseases are relatively complex chronic medical and nursing problems and will be considered briefly as a group.

Two general types of neuromuscular difficulty may develop: (1) neuromuscular function may be depressed causing weakness, or (2) neuromuscular function may be exaggerated causing spasm, tremors or rigidity in movement. Each type has many variations, and each is associated with weakness, fatigue and difficulty in muscular performance, often with complete disability. The spasm of the muscle is often also associated with pain. Sometimes these conditions come as the result of a known cause which can be treated specifically, but the more common and important neuromuscular diseases have no known cause and offer a poor prognosis for recovery. Fortunately for the patient, treatment with fair relief is more common today than ever before.

The common conditions which belong to this group are myasthenia gravis, poliomyelitis, Parkinson's disease, rheumatic disease, low back syndrome, torticollis (stiff neck), frozen shoulder syndrome, fibrositis, hemiplegia. In some of these conditions the muscle spasm is secondary to the fundamental condition.

Weakness of Movement

For weakness and diffculty in movement due to neuromuscular disease the drugs used act mainly on the transmission of impulses between nerve and muscle. In the treatment of myasthenia gravis, neostigmine (or physostigmine) may be used. At one time ephedrine was also used in this condition. Quinine has also been reported to be of value, and recently isoflurophate (fluropryl, DFP) has been advised. All of these drugs exert an effect on the parasympathetic nervous system, but they also exert an influence on the transmission or conduction of impulses from nerve to muscle.

Spasm

In the spasm of neuromuscular disorders, treatment depends on the cause of the disease and whether the spasm is a primary or secondary manifestation. Obviously the most reasonable way to treat the condition is by curing the primary disease. Unfortunately, this is rarely possible with drugs. In poliomyelitis, for example, muscle spasm causes excruciating pain. The spasm is due to the disease in the spinal cord. The spinal cord disease is not affected by drugs or physical devices. The spasm must, therefore, be treated in the muscle rather than in the spinal cord. Physiotherapy may be helpful. The hot packs of Sister Kenney provide relaxation, and other physical methods may also be beneficial. Such relaxation prevents the shortening of the muscle which often causes permanent deformity after the disease has been cured. The most effective muscle relaxant is curare or pharmacologically related drugs which block the neuromuscular junction and produce a partial or complete paralysis of muscles. The effects of curare-like drugs are rather intense, cause great weakness and in large doses may stop breathing. While they are being used, the patient requires constant and close attention.

Tremors and Rigidity

Tremors and rigidity of movement which make locomotion and other coordinated movements gross and unskilled are also found in the neuromuscular disorders. Such rigidity and tremors of Parkinson's disease may be helped by mephenesin and trihexylphenidyl (artane). When these drugs are used the patient must be carefully watched for side actions, which are both common and disagreeable.

Drugs Used in Treatment of Musculo-Skeletal Disorders

Analgesics (nonaddicting)   Autonomics
Antiarthritics   Hormones
Antibiotics   Relaxants

Study Questions

1. What group of drugs is frequently employed in the treatment of muscle and joint pain? What are toxic signs and symptoms?

2. Neostigmine may be used as a diagnostic test or as treatment in myasthenia gravis. What are its actions in relation to this disease? What special responsibilities does the nurse have in relation to the availability of such a drug?

3. What group of drugs is used in the relief of severe muscle spasm to produce relaxation?

21

TREATMENT OF BLOOD DYSCRASIAS

Although blood is a liquid, its functions are varied and important, and it should be thought of as one of the vital organs. Its functions have been described as follows:

1. *Respiration:* Blood brings oxygen from the lungs to cells and removes carbon dioxide. Without blood there is cellular asphyxia.

2. *Nutrition*: Blood brings nutriment from the digestive organs to all cells of the body; without blood there is cellular starvation.

3. *Excretion*: Blood carries the products of cellular activity (uric acid, urea, creatinine, etc.) from the cells to the kidneys. Without blood, cells are poisoned by their own waste products.

4. *Communication*: Blood carries hormones from organs producing them to other organs using them, thus assisting in the hormonal regulation on the activity of the body; changes in the hormonal composition of blood stimulate or depress respiration, heart rate, blood pressure and so forth. Without blood the various organs of the body are isolated.

5. *Defense*: Blood brings white blood cells, antibodies and other defense materials to infected and injured parts of the body. Without blood the body is without defense.

6. *Temperature regulation*: The circulating blood, as described on page 126, equalizes the temperature of the body, and maintains the equilibrium by conserving the body heat or accelerating its loss through skin radiation. Without blood there is no temperature regulation.

Plasma

Approximately half of the volume of blood is comprised of a fluid called plasma; the rest is made up of the formed elements,

242

blood cells and platelets. Plasma is a yellowish fluid which contains about 6 per cent of protein and fibrinogen, a material which forms a blood clot when blood stands. The blood proteins are comprised of several fractions, of which the alpha globulins, in particular, contain most of the specific antibodies against disease. Blood proteins provide the blood with a buffering power and with osmotic tension. In addition to the proteins plasma contains metabolites, such as urea, uric acid, creatinine, carbon dioxide, hormones and food elements, fat globules, sugar, protein, minerals, vitamins, electrolyte. In the main, the blood merely serves as the vehicle to carry these products from one part of the body to another.

Formed Elements

The formed elements of the blood, the white and red blood cells and platelets, have different functions. The function of red blood cells and the red pigment (hemoglobin) inside of them is to carry oxygen from the lungs to the cells; the white blood cells are part of the defenses of the body against irritation, injury and infection; the function of the platelet is to start the blood clotting process.

Excessive amounts of blood place a burden on the heart; too little produces shock. Body fluids must therefore be kept normal in quantity as well as in composition. In most instances of blood dyscrasias there is no alteration in blood fluid composition. Low blood protein is sometimes the consequence of blood loss, sometimes of chronic infection, sometimes of continued albuminuria. In the main, these may be corrected by intravenous (or even oral) administration of the needed materials. The simplest way to provide these when the need is urgent is by whole blood or plasma transfusions. Other chemical constituents of the blood may be abnormal as a consequence of disease. These are best replaced by the use of the so-called parenteral fluids (page 144).

Nature of Blood Dyscrasias

Blood dyscrasias usually consist of abnormalities in the formed elements rather than in the composition of the plasma. One or more of these formed constituents of blood may be abnormal, either in character or in amount; thus they may be defective, deficient or excessive. Each type of abnormality, in turn, produces its own kind of disturbance or symptom.

Abnormalities in composition of blood may be secondary to some other disease; these are the so-called secondary disturbances. Thus the white cell count rises in some infections while in others it may go down. In allergic conditions the eosinophiles, a particular type of white cell may increase. In some chronic infections the hemoglobin content of blood may fall, or after chronic bleeding there may be an anemia. The anemias with known cause are secondary anemias and are usually rectified when the primary disease is cured.

There is also a series of disturbances in the composition of the formed elements of the blood, in which the primary site of the disease appears to be in the blood forming organ, the bone marrow, or in some aspect of blood formation; these are the so-called primary disturbances. In most instances the cause of such primary disease is not known, although recently knowledge of some of these has come to light. Some of these dyscrasias are found to be the result of a type of intoxication. In general, bone marrow function seems to be highly susceptible to the effects of drugs and poisons. The primary blood dyscrasias are generally of greater seriousness than secondary disturbances of blood composition, perhaps because no cause is known for the primary type and, therefore, no real cure possible.

There are many types of medicaments which are used in the treatment of both the primary and the secondary types of blood dyscrasias: (1) stimulants to hemoglobin formation, (2) stimulants and depressants of white cell formation, (4) stimulants and depressants of the blood clotting mechanism, (5) replacements of materials necessary for the maturation of red blood cells.

Hemoglobin

Hemoglobin is concerned with the transportation of oxygen to the cells from the lungs; if hemoglobin is deficient for any reason, and the defect is serious enough, a certain degree of cellular asphyxia results. As a consequence we find weakness and fatiguability in a case of anemia. Anemia may be due to blood loss, systemic or local infections, or primary disease of the blood forming system. When anemia is due to blood loss, whatever the cause, the use of substantial doses of iron, providing the bleeding has ceased, is likely to be followed by satisfactory results. Other metals may also be helpful but these are needed in such small amounts that they are usually present as impurities in the iron or are in food, and are not needed as a separate medication.

There are practical aspects to the use of iron. Since it must be given in relatively large doses, it is not usually possible to administer it by injection, and the oral route must be used instead. Iron salts tend to upset the stomach, especially in the large doses needed. For this reason it is well to take precautions to avoid gastro-intestinal difficulties. Most patients tolerate iron better when they take it immediately after eating. Some find that they can build up a tolerance to iron if they start with small doses, building up to larger ones in a few days. In general, ferrous salts of iron are more tolerable than ferric salts, although there is little practical difference in effectiveness. The most common iron salt now used is ferrous sulfate; some patients, however, find ferrous gluconate easier to retain. It is well to warn all patients who take iron medication that it tends to turn the stools a dark green or black; some patients not appraised of this may be frightened by the appearance of the stool.

Red Blood Cells

Red blood cells, so colored by the hemoglobin which they contain, are formed in the bone marrow, but for maturation, they require absorption by the stomach. This is accomplished with the aid of extrinsic factors (essential elements in the diet) and intrinsic factors (products of normal liver function). Disturbances or deficiencies in any of these may result in seriously reduced numbers of red cells, defective red cells or excessive destruction of red cells. In addition, chronic infections and toxemias may depress red cell formation.

Primary anemias, with an insufficient number as well as defective red cells, are often serious diseases, the best known of which is pernicious anemia (Addison's disease). This is a complex ailment due largely to a defect in red cell maturation and can often be helped, but not cured, by the use of such materials as liver, liver extracts, stomach extracts, folic acid, vitamin B_{12}. It is not at all helped by iron. It is important to treat such primary anemias because one of the secondary effects is a serious and irreversible alteration in the spinal cord which produces weakness and paralysis.

Red cell formation which is sometimes excessive may be due to physiologic stimulation produced by low oxygen content of blood, e.g., high altitudes, low oxygen content in the air, chronic heart and pulmonary disease in which the blood is not well ventilated by the lungs. One of the diseases of excessive red cell formation is polycythemia vera from which serious consequences may develop. There is no known cure for this disease but it may be helped by blood letting or by the use of drugs (radio-phosphorus, phenyl-hydrazine) which depress the blood formation. Such toxic drugs are also dangerous drugs; they must be used with great caution and the patient watched assiduously.

White Blood Cells

White blood cells are part of the defenses of the blood, and usually increase in number in the bloodstream in most infections, and increase in number as well, at the site of an injury. In diseases such as leukopenia in which the number is seriously depressed, the patient's life may be imperiled. For this reason, a drug which would stimulate their production would be a most useful material. The only materials which were supposed to have such an action were the pento-nucleotides, but the property of these agents is questioned by most hematologists and the drug is now rarely used. In the case of serious depression of the white cells, in addition to attacking the cause of white cell depression, the present practice is to provide the patient with drug defense against infection in the form of large doses of penicillin and other antibiotic materials. Blood transfusions also provide support. Unless recovery occurs spontaneously the ultimate outlook is dismal.

The leukemias, acute and chronic, are a group of diseases in which the number of white cells is enormously increased. In many respects they resemble a malignant tumor of the white cells. Leukemias as a disease group are well known; treatment of each type is somewhat different.

The acute form of leukemia runs a devastatingly short course against which little is effective, except, in some instances, cortisone and corticotropin (ACTH). Neither cures the disease but the life of the patient seems to be prolonged when they are used. Many other drugs such as the folic acid antagonists have been tried but most of them with too little effect to consider here.

The chronic form of leukemia may continue for many years. At first the white cell count is easily depressed by a number of drugs, arsenicals, nitrogen mustards, radio-phosphorus, as well as by x-ray and radium. It seems to make little difference which is used first, but after a period of time the disease becomes resistant and the treatment with any of them becomes ineffectual.

Bleeding and Blood Clotting

There are many conditions in which the tendency to bleeding is so great that spontaneous and sometimes serious hemorrhage tends to occur. Hemophilia, purpura and severe liver damage are a few conditions in which excessive bleeding occurs. There are others in which there is an exaggerated tendency for blood to clot, with serious symptoms resulting from the intravascular clots; such diseases as thrombo-phlebitis and thrombo-angiitis obliterans. The diseases with bleeding tendency may sometimes be effectively treated by operation (splenectomy). In other instances temporary relief may be provided with whole blood transfusions, vitamin K (or equivalents) and local application of fibrin foam and astringent drugs.

Anticoagulants

The anticoagulants are drugs which inhibit the blood clotting mechanism. Heparin and dicumarol (and related drugs) are anticoagulants used to prevent intravascular blood clotting in such diseases as thrombophlebitis and coronary infarction, and to prevent the more serious complications of thromboembolization. In some cases of mitral stenosis, the disease is marked by occasional or frequent showers of emboli. These can be prevented by depressing the blood clotting mechanism. It is to be remembered, however, that the drugs do not dissolve clots which are already present and that the clots already formed may break off and cause serious embolization even though anticoagulants have been given in effective doses; anticoagulants, at best, merely prevent the further growth of thrombi.

The program of depressing the clotting mechanism has hazards and should not be undertaken by one without experience and laboratory facilities for following the course of medication. It is possible to depress clotting to the extent that serious internal hemorrhage occurs. This emergency requires prompt treatment with blood transfusion or vitamin K.

The proper dosage of anticoagulant is determined by a continuous type of therapeutic experimentation, in which the dose for a day is determined by the effect of the preceding day's dose. Thus, such drugs may not be used unless laboratory facilities for regular determination of prothrombin time are available.

Drugs Used in Treatment of Blood Dyscrasias

Antianemics	Hematinics, *see* antianemics
Anticoagulants	Hemostatics
Antimitotics	Hormones
Bone marrow depressants	Parenteral fluids
Coagulants, *see* Hemostatics	Radioactive phosphorus

Study Questions

1. Indicate and describe some of the functions of the blood.

2. What are the constituents of blood and the functions of each?

3. What factors should be considered by the nurse in regard to the administration of iron preparations to patients?

4. Why, in the use of anticoagulant therapy, may drugs such as heparin and dicumarol be administered at the same time?

5. Why are doses of these drugs ordered each day, early in the course of therapy?

6. What are the nurse's responsibilities in relation to the observation of patients receiving anticoagulant therapy?

7. What drugs and measures are taken to relieve toxic signs of these drugs?

22

TREATMENT OF NEOPLASTIC DISEASES

The outstanding characteristic of neoplastic diseases, otherwise called newgrowths or tumors, is the tendency of certain groups of cells to increase in size. In the full-grown adult, all cells normally multiply slowly and at a rate approximately equal to that of the wearing out of old cells so that no growth or enlargement results. But in neoplastic disease some cells increase in number far beyond the needs for replacement so that growth in a particular spot or part of an organ goes on at an unusual rate and an enlargement or tumor develops. Thus, in a tumor or newgrowth of the thyroid gland, there is an excessive number of thyroid cells; in a tumor of the prostate there are too many prostate cells. Comparable situations develop in the blood-forming organs, an excessive number of red blood cells leads to a condition known as polycythemia and an excessive number of white blood cells causes leukemia.

Symptoms in neoplastic disease may develop from the excessive function of the enlarged organ, from the pressure the mass exerts by its abnormal size on the organs adjoining it, or from the fact that the unnecessary cells act more or less as parasites drawing on the rest of the body for their nutrition but contributing nothing to the well-being of the body.

A distinction may be drawn between malignant and benign tumors. The growth of a benign tumor is restrained and it remains localized; a malignant tumor is relatively unrestrained and, eventually, tumor cells leave the site of origin and set up sites of new growth in distant parts of the body. These emigrations are known as metastases. The development of metastatic growths in vital organs, and the drain on body economy by many of them diffusely spread over the body, are the properties of the malignant growth which eventually kill the patient.

The reasons for the excessive multiplication of cells and the formation of tumors are unknown; in some cases irritation or hormonal defects may contribute, but in general, there is no adequate explanation. In most cases, therefore, treatment cannot be directed against the cause. Since the fundamental characteristic, as already mentioned, is the excessive multiplication (mitosis) of cells, palliative treatment is directed against this aspect of cellular activity. Most of the drugs used are, therefore, the so-called antimitotics.

The symptoms of neoplastic diseases depend largely on three factors: (1) the physical effects of the actual bulk of the tumor, exerting an unusual amount of pressure; (2) the draining effects of the parasitism of the tumor cells on the body; (3) disturbances of certain functions of the involved organs. Thus there may be severe pain when a tumor presses against a nerve trunk or against a sensitive organ, there may be serious emaciation as the result of the invasion of the body by the spreading new growths, and there may be special symptoms due to disturbed activity of a tumor-ridden organ.

Surgery and X-Ray

Surgical treatment consists of removing the tumor. The disease may be completely and permanently eradicated by surgical removal in the case of benign tumors and early malignant growths. Once the disease has spread from the site of its origin, it can no longer be considered a localized disease and, therefore, it is no longer possible to cure it surgically. In some cases it may be possible to destroy the tumor in situations by the use of x-ray or radium, and when this measure does not cure the condition it may alleviate it. These latter modalities are physical antimitotic procedures tending to inhibit the activity of multiplying cells.

Medical Treatment

In instances in which surgery and x-ray cannot offer relief, medical measures may be tried. It may be stated that, at the time of this writing there are no medical measures for the treatment of malignant tumors which frequently hold any hope of cure. At best they are palliative measures. In any event, often the relief they give is outstanding, and there are rare instances of cures. The benefits they have over surgery and x-ray is their availability for use in the home and in areas in which radium or the high-voltage equipment for deep x-ray therapy is not available.

The drugs used in the specific treatment of cancer may be grouped as follows: (1) hormones, (2) antimitotic drugs, (3) radioactive drugs and (4) miscellaneous drugs. These drugs are not commonly used in treatment of the benign type of neoplastic diseases in which surgery is almost always a certain measure. They are used with malignant tumors, only when surgery seems futile, and when x-ray or radium are not desirable, practicable, or available.

Hormones

There is evidence that cancer of the prostate gland in the male, and cancer of the breast in the female, are responsive to castration and treatment with the sex hormones. In these conditions, even when the cancer has spread to other parts of the body there may be dramatic improvement from the use of the proper hormone in adequate dosage. Unfortunately, sooner or later the condition ceases to respond to the hormone and continues its relentless course. But in the interim, the patient may improve to the extent that life again becomes enjoyable and he can pursue useful work. Since these drugs do not promise a cure, they are never substituted for surgery when the latter offers any hope. In general, the sex hormones of the opposite sex are used and, in some cases, they are used in combination with castration. Thus, for breast cancer, androgenic drugs such as testosterone may be given the female patient, while for cancer of the prostate, estrogenic drugs are given to the male patient. In the case of females over 60 with cancer of the breast, the estrogenic hormones may also be useful. In general, rather large doses are administered, so large that in the male, symptoms of effeminism, and in the female, symptoms of virilism, often appear.

Antimitotic Drugs

X-rays and radium produce their effects on neoplasms by inhibiting mitosis or cell multiplication, thereby preventing further growth. In the case of very sensitive tumors, the mass may disappear. In general, actively multiplying cells are more sensitive to the effects of x-ray and radium than are normal and slowly dividing cells. For this reason when these modalities are applied to an area which contains both cancerous and normal cells, they depress the cancerous tissue more intensively than the normal. But they do, nonetheless, also affect normal tissues, sometimes seriously, frequently tending to produce disagreeable side effects.

A relatively new group of drugs used in the treatment of some forms of cancer are the nitrogen mustards. These drugs are antimitotic and their effects on actively dividing cells are similar to those of x-ray and radium. Therefore, the same generalizations about results also apply. Antimitotic drugs in general are systemic poisons and are likely to produce serious toxic effects unless carefully watched. They are especially prone to have depressant effects on bone marrow and blood formation. Some malignancies which seem to be more susceptible to the nitrogen mustards than others include Hodgkin's disease, chronic leukemias, polycythemia, multiple myeloma, lymphosarcoma, lung cancers.

Radioactive Drugs

Radioactive drugs, those treated in an atomic pile, form a new and highly interesting group of drugs. Their special virtues lie in the fact that they not only exert an antimitotic action identical to that of x-ray and radium, but also that in some instances after internal administration, these effects can be exerted on a particular organ without danger of injuring other tissues of the body.

Unfortunately, however, their practical value in the treatment of cancer is distinctly limited, and in general, there is more academic than practical interest in them. There are a few exceptions. The most important of all is radioiodine (I^{131}) in the treatment of cancer of the thyroid gland. Since this gland always extracts iodine from the blood, it will extract radioiodine in the same manner and concentrate it in the gland. As a consequence, mitosis in the gland is inhibited by this radioactive material in much the same way as it is inhibited when the gland is irritated by x-ray. However, this treatment may not be as effective in thyroid cancer as in hyperthyroidism because cancer cells do not usually concentrate radioiodine with the same intensity as functioning cells.

On the same basis, radiophosphorus is given in some blood dyscrasias, and radiocobalt in other forms of cancer. The results are not so frequently encouraging to make this the treatment of choice and already it has given way to other simpler and more dependable methods of providing relief.

Other activated drugs may be introduced into medicine for similar purposes and certain generalizations may be made which apply to all. Radioactive elements and drugs can be useful only if they are concentrated by the neoplastic (as against the normal) cells; otherwise, the radiation effects will be produced throughout the body. To be useful, the radioactive drug must have a period of activity long enough to exert a real therapeutic effect but not so long that activity continues to the point of danger.

There are also many technical difficulties which seriously limit the extent of their usefulness. These are present in judging dose, handling and administering the radioactive drugs.

Miscellaneous Drugs

Stilbamidine has been reported of value in the relief of pain and symptoms of multiple myeloma but with no arrest of the course of the disease. It is thought that this drug works by selective penetration into the abnormal cells. Serious neurologic reactions have been reported and its usefulness is limited.

Folic acid antagonists such as amino-teropterin, aminopterin, adenopterin and methopterin have been used in leukemia and other forms of incurable cancer. Relief has been reported by some observers but no cures. These drugs may cause serious toxic symptoms and must be watched carefully. On the other hand, many patients have been treated daily with these drugs for over a year without symptoms of toxicity. These are still "experimental drugs."

Cortisone and corticotropin (ACTH) have been used with dramatic improvement in children with acute leukemias, a condition completely resistant to all other forms of therapy. The length of the remissions induced with these drugs is variable, but rarely for a significant period. There are indications that these drugs may also be used in other related conditions such as the lymphomatous malignancies after they have developed resistance to other forms of therapy.

Among the long list of other drugs tried and discarded, but still occasionally heard from are Coley's mixed bacterial toxins, Shear's polysacharides, urine extracts, virus therapy, ACS (antireticular cytotoxic serum), K-R, meylokentric acid, vitamins, biotin, pyridoxin, dyes and enzyme poisons. The list of drugs which have failed is long indeed.

Palliative and pain-relieving drugs are used extensively in the treatment of the final and painful stages of cancer. These present special problems in the relief of pain which is discussed elsewhere and which often justifies the deliberate induction of drug addiction.

Drugs Used in Treatment of Neoplastic Diseases

Androgens	Estrogens
Anticarcinogenics	Hormones
Antimitotics, *see* Anticarcinogenics	Radioactive Drugs

Study Questions

1. What do we mean by antimitotic drugs? Give examples.

2. What major factors determine the symptoms of neoplastic diseases?

3. For the treatment of what specific neoplasms are hormones used? Give examples.

4. What is one of the greatest dangers which may result from the use of antimitotic drugs? What precautions are taken to recognize this during the course of therapy?

5. What special advantages do radioactive drugs have in the treatment of neoplastic disease? Give examples.

23

TREATMENT OF SKIN DISORDERS

The skin is a complex and important organ which functions to protect the tissues beneath from injury, irritation, infection and invasion. At the same time it is a responsive sensory organ and appreciative of many sensations: pain, itching, tingling, burning, hot and cold, pin-prick and two-point discrimination. As an organ it is capable of a variety of expressions in the form of symptoms, pain, itching, tingling, eruptions, color changes, swellings, blisters, postules, bullae and hives. The list of skin diseases is long and in a great many cases the cause is unknown. They may be due to irritation, allergies, infection, injuries, congenital defects, degenerative diseases, malignancies, drug reactions, intoxications, hormonal disturbances and emotional crises. Treatment is most effective when directed specifically against the cause of the skin disorder, but often this cannot be done. Skin symptoms are not only disagreeable to look at but can also be profoundly disturbing, so much so that in unrelieved intense itching a patient may attempt suicide. In addition, there are many serious skin diseases which drain one's health and there are some which are fatal.

Relief of Skin Symptoms

Skin symptoms may be relieved by a large variety of medications, sometimes requiring considerable trial and error before the proper one for the particular condition is discovered. Some of them are briefly considered below.

Emmolients are drugs used to sooth the skin.

Caustics are chemicals used to destroy or burn away diseased portions of the skin.

Antiseptics are used to destroy or inhibit micro-organisms on the surface of the skin. It is to be remembered that the skin itself has good defenses against the common micro-organisms, and that chemical disinfectants may destroy these natural agents. Relatively strong antiseptic agents may be used when the skin is prepared for an operation and when the surgeon cleanses his hands. These are applied together with soap for a considerable period of time, and even when this is efficiently done, the skin is not completely disinfected. Cleanliness of the skin is an important approach to skin disinfection.

Surface anesthetics are used to relieve skin symptoms. In this instance, the type of local anesthetic which is absorbed from the surface of the skin must be chosen, the common local anesthetic, procaine (novocaine) for example, will not work when applied locally but drugs such as ethyl aminobenzoate (benzocaine) and tetracaine are absorbed from the skin and may be used effectively for surface anesthesia.

Astringents are materials which tend to contract the surface of the skin.

Styptics are strong astringents which are capable of closing small gaps in the skin and stopping superficial bleeding.

Desquamating and keratolytic agents are drugs which peel off the outer layers of the skin. These are used in an attempt to peel off a diseased area.

Epithelializers are drugs used to encourage the repair of the skin over wounds. The action of most drugs used for this purpose is questionable. In most instances it is probable that these drugs are protective and in that way only aid in epithelization.

Antihistaminic and other antiallergic drugs are commonly used in allergic disorders of the skin (page 132). When the allergy is especially acute or resistant to treatment cortisone and corticotropin are also used (page 135).

Metabolic drugs of a variety of kinds are used today for some of the skin eruptions in which it is felt that the eruption is due to a metabolic disorder. Chief and most common among these is psoriasis. For the treatment of this resistant condition many drugs with systemic and metabolic actions are used, most common of which are the lipotropic agents such as choline, methionine and inositol.

Itch

Itching is the outstanding dermatologic symptom. It varies in intensity from a mild itch to one which is devastating. Severe and continued itching may sometimes drive a patient to suicide, but more commonly it is only an annoyance and a source of embarassment.

The treatment of itch depends on its nature, cause and the pathologic condition associated with it. If possible the cause should be eliminated. In a number of instances, however, it may be essential to relieve the itching regardless of the treatment of the underlying disease.

There are a number of palliative measures for this purpose. Among them are the surface anesthetics, and emolients or demulcents. These agents are applied topically in the form of ointments, paints, pastes, solutions and washes. In severe relentless itching, procaine may be injected intravenously. In itching due to allergy the antihistaminic drugs may be helpful.

Skin Antisepsis

As already explained there are serious limitations to the degree to which local antisepsis may be obtained. In many skin infections, since the infection is superficial, logic may suggest the use of a local antiseptic, but often the use of such an agent may aggravate instead of help a skin lesion. There are conditions, however, in which such measures may assist in the cure, or at least prevent the extension of the infection to adjacent areas of skin. It is important that drugs used for this purpose be so dilute that they will not damage the healthy or irritate the diseased skin. The list of local antiseptics is long and the choice of the drugs depends on the nature of the infecting organism.

Drugs Used in Treatment of Skin Disorders

Allergenic extracts	Antihistaminics
Anesthetics (surface)	Antipruritics
Antibiotics	Antiseptics (local)

Astringents

Caustics

Chemotherapeutics

Corrosives, *see* Caustics

Demulcents

Deodorants

Depilatories

Detergents

Emolients, *see* Demulcents

Epilators, *see* Depilatories

Hormones

Keratolytics

Protectives, *see* Demulcents

Rubifacients

Vesicants

Study Questions

1. Indicate some of the causes of skin diseases and some of their manifestations.

2. What important factors should the nurse be aware of in relation to the use of disinfectants on the skin?

24

TREATMENT OF MEDICAL EMERGENCIES

The nurse stands in a critical position in respect to all medical emergencies. On the one hand, she is usually the first to appreciate that the patient's condition is taking a critical turn, while on the other hand she is not always in a position to apply the proper drugs either because she does not have the authority or because she does not have the training. Yet the fact remains that in a number of medical emergencies if the nurse were in a position to treat at once, the patient's life might be spared or prolonged. Many physicians anticipate the emergencies which are possible and leave orders for medications to be used should such situations develop.

From the nurse's point of view, medical emergencies may be divided into three groups: (1) those in which the situation is so critical that unless the proper procedure is immediately applied the patient may die, (2) those in which there is sufficient time to contact the doctor and get instructions from him and (3) those in which there is enough time to wait for the doctor to arrive to direct the proceedings. Fortunately for everyone concerned, most emergencies fall into the third category.

The most urgent emergencies are those in which poisoning, hemorrhage, asphyxia (suffocation) or shock occurs. An extensive discussion of poison follows. The hemorrhage may be internal or external, due to trauma or disease. Asphyxia may be due to a variety of causes ranging from physical suffocation to smoke, poisonous fumes, intoxications, heart failure, pleural effusions, anemia, pneumonia and tuberculosis. Shock may be due to trauma, poisoning, hemorrhage, coronary infarction, pulmonary embolism or serious infection.

259

There are, in addition, many other medical situations which require prompt attention. Most emergent situations are surgical and traumatic but some are purely medical. The treatment of these various conditions is considered in the several sections of this book; further detailing of treatment cannot be given here. The Materia Medica lists many antidotes in the sections on the drugs against which they may be used. The nurse, in the home or on the ward, should be prepared as well as possible to provide immediately the materials and drugs which are needed for the treatment of such emergencies as they arise.

Drugs Used in Medical Emergencies

In each illness some (but not all) of the emergency possibilities may be anticipated and provided for. In general, however, it is always well to be provided with a kit for the most common medical emergencies. A list of drugs which should be included in such a kit, together with a concise indication of the purpose of each, is given in table 4. It may be noted that there are adequate substitutes for many of the drugs listed in this table. The instruments necessary to administer the drugs in the emergency kit cannot be considered here, but obviously, means must be provided for the proper application.

Poisoning

The results in treating serious cases of poisoning are usually unsatisfactory. Whether the poisoning be deliberate or accidental, suicidal, or homicidal, it is often discovered or diagnosed too late for successful treatment. To complicate matters still further, events may take a sudden and unexpected turn in the course of poisoning, and a patient who seems to be in good condition may abruptly change into one who is critically ill and whose needs for effective therapy are most urgent. There is still another complication of poisoning which makes its treatment so discouraging; there are cases in which a patient in deep coma or shock is treated for effects of the poison with apparent success and who survives the direct affects of the poison, only to die later of a secondary effect. In many such cases death is due to kidney failure resulting from prolonged shock or from hypostatic pneumonia due to log-like coma

Table 4—Drugs Which Should Be Included in a Medical Emergency Kit

Emergency	Drug
Acid burns	Sodium bicarbonate
Alkali burns	Dulute acetic acid
Alkaloid poisoning	Potassium permanganate
Allergic crises	Cortisone
Anesthesia	Ether
Anesthesia, local	Procaine
Anesthesia, surface (eye, skin or mucous membrane)	Tetracaine
Anginal pain	Amyl nitrite
Antiallergic	Epinephrine
Antihistaminic	Diphenhydramine
Antispasmodic	Atropine, Aminophyllin
Asphyxia	Oxygen
Barbiturate poisoning	Picrotoxin
Bleeding	Vitamin K
Burns	Cortisone
Cardiac stimulant	Digitoxin, Ouabain
Cerebral stimulant	Caffeine
Circulatory stimulant	Epinephrine, Nikethamide, Hydroxyamphetamine
Dehydration	Saline
Diabetic coma	Insulin
Diuretic	Meralluride
Emetic	Apomorphine
Excitement, anxiety	Pentobarbital, Amobarbital
Insulin shock	Dextrose
Infections	Sulfadiazine, Penicillin
Infections, superficial	Tincture of iodine
Metal poisoning	Dimercaprol
Migraine headache	Ergotamine
Pain	Morphine, Codeine
Shock	Plasma
Strychnine poisoning	Ether
Thrombophlebitis	Dicumarol
Uterine bleeding	Ergotrate, Testosterone
Wounds, contaminated	Tetanus antitoxin

for too long a period of time. There are very few conditions in medicine in which prompt diagnosis and precise treatment so frequently mean the difference between life and death.

Poisoning is a medical condition in which the first person on the scene, whoever he may be and whatever his training, is the one who is in a position to do the most good. The possibility of poisoning must be borne in mind in all cases of unexplained coma or even chronic illness. It is proper to point out that the possibility of poisoning is not frequently prominent in the conscious thinking of nurses and doctors. As a result there are very few cases of homicidal poisoning for example, in which the symptoms are recognized or the condition diagnosed before the postmortem examination.

The treatment of poisoning may be divided into three categories listed in the usual order of their importance to the patient and his survival: (1) recognition of the fact of poisoning, (2) prompt institution of the general measures for treatment of poisoning, (3) application of antidotes specific for the poison in the particular case. The specific antidote is the least important and in fact there is none in many cases.

Diagnosis of Poisoning

Since early diagnosis is so vital, the suspicion of poisoning by the nurse may be the critical event in the patient's life. Only a small proportion of suicidal poisonings make any direct announcement of the fact by letter, note or other evidence; the majority of poisoning cases require diagnosis. Poisoning may result from accident such as: (1) taking of mislabeled drugs, (2) the misreading of the labels on drugs (especially at night when a sleepy patient may take medication to relieve some form of distress), (3) accidental overdosage (too large a dose or too frequently taken), (4) hypersensitivity or idiosyncracies, (5) accidental exposure in industry. Poisoning may also be deliberate, as in cases of homicide or suicide.

The state of intoxication in which the patient is found may be early or late, mild or intense, but the fact that the symptoms of poisoning are not serious at the time of diagnosis does not mean that the state of poisoning will not continue to progress into one which takes the patient's life. All cases of poisoning must be treated as serious ones until it has been determined that less than a fatal dose of the poison remains in the patient's system.

Poisoning may be suspected in all persons with unexplained symptoms who are taking drugs, in cases in which symptoms appear suddenly without medical explanation, in all cases of unexplained unconsciousness, in patients having convulsions who are known not to be epileptics and in undiagnosed illnesses appearing in a number of related or associated patients at approximately the same time (a small epidemic of undiagnosed illness.)

The possibility of suicidal poisoning should be considered in all unconscious patients who are known to have unstable personalities, with serious business or marital difficulties, or a history of a previous attempt at suicide. Young people more frequently attempt suicide than older ones. A note, an empty bottle or an empty syringe may be found near the patient to give the telling clue, but too often these are not present at the bedside. The pockets of the clothing may be emptied for drug containers; since the bathroom is often used as the site of the taking the drug it should be examined for evidences of poison. If a bottle is found, the prescription number on it may provide the simplest way of finding the pharmacist who filled it and what the bottle contained. At the same time be certain also to find out the number of pills or capsules which were originally contained in the bottle. Note the posture of the patient's body, look for automatic or convulsive movements and examine the body for the puncture marks of an injection even if an empty syringe is not found.

If the patient is still conscious there is a possibility that he will inform you he has taken poison either accidentally or deliberately. Never dismiss such statements until they are proved to be untrue; always take them seriously and proceed as if they were true.

It is an interesting point that there are fashions in suicidal and homicidal poisoning and that many people will use a drug which has received considerable newspaper publicity. At the present time the barbiturates are in fashion for the taking of one's own life.

General Measures

Have someone call the doctor at once. While waiting for his instructions apply measures to remove all the unabsorbed poison from the stomach and prevent or slow up its absorption. If the poison has been injected, nothing can be done along these lines. The longer the period between the taking of the poison and emptying of the stomach, the less benefit that may come from this procedure, since absorption continues as times goes on. Speed is of the greatest importance here and if many hours have elapsed since the poison was taken, little benefit can be expected from emptying the stomach.

Emesis

The quickest way for the nurse to empty the stomach is to induce vomiting. In the case of an unconscious patient this is not easy to accomplish, and even if emesis can be induced, there is grave danger of aspiration pneumonia from this procedure. If the patient is already in coma, it may be presumed that most of the drug has already been absorbed and the nurse should, therefore, wait for the doctor to advise how to empty the stomach. The unconscious patient may be placed in a supine position in bed and his head should be hung over the edge of the bed below his recumbent body to prevent the aspiration of stomach contents.

In the conscious patient the quickest way to induce vomiting is by rubbing the back of the pharynx with the index finger. The nurse's finger should be stuck well back into the patient's mouth until it reaches the back of the pharynx and then the pharynx should be tickled. There are household emetics such as powdered English mustard (not the usual American mustard which comes made up in jars). This is rarely in the kitchen and if present, it is difficult to find. It may turn out to be too old to be effective and in the end it is not always dependable. Sirup of ipecac (1 teaspoonful) may induce vomiting but few people keep this medication at home. A subcutaneous injection of apomorphine (5 mg.) can be depended upon to induce prompt and violent emesis but this must be prescribed by the doctor. Old solutions of apomorphine may be ineffective.

Gastric lavage, using a relatively large bore stomach tube, is the most effective and dependable means of emptying the stomach but such equipment is not usually found around the home, which is the common site for suicidal attempts. Thus the finger remains the simplest and the most readily available means of inducing vomiting promptly. Chemicals such as zinc or copper sulfate should not be used by the nurse as emetics without specific orders from the physician.

It must be borne in mind that violent emesis is a strenuous act the nature of which should be taken into especial consideration with the very sick patient. After the stomach is emptied the first time the patient may be permitted to drink some milk, water, tea or other bland fluid, and the vomiting can be again induced. This will tend to wash the stomach. If this is accomplished without much distress it can be repeated several times.

Delaying Absorption

The absorption of poisons often can be delayed by food, and, for this reason, poison taken on an empty stomach is a more serious matter than poison taken after meals. Eggs and milk are not only readily available foods in most households, but they are also among the most effective foods for delaying absorption. Fortunately, virtually any other food will also have this kind of effect. It is a wise precaution, therefore, to give the patient milk, eggs, an eggnog or some food to retain even after his stomach has been emptied.

Respiration

Respiration is a matter of great importance. Poor oxygenation of blood due to depressed respiration or mucus plugging of the trachea or bronchi may produce serious damage to brain and other vital organs. Usually this is more of a problem and requires greater attention in the unconscious patient who cannot indicate his distress or cough to remove mucus than in the conscious patient. The nurse should note the color of the skin and mucous membranes, the rate and depth of respiration, the presence of frothy saliva and she should listen for the noisy breathing indicative of mucus obstruction in the tracheo-bronchial tree. She can help the patient with respiratory distress by extending his head, by sucking out mucus and applying artificial respiration if spontaneous respiration is seriously depressed.

Coma and Shock

In patients who have been in coma for a long period of time there is the serious possibility of hypostatic pneumonia. Antibiotics are now given routinely to prevent this complication. In seriously poisoned patients the state of shock may eventually cause irreversible kidney damage. Often the kidney damage of this type makes its appearance after considerable delay, in some cases after the patient apparently has recovered. The prompt treatment of shock is, therefore, a vital element in the treatment of poisoning. Signs of circulatory collapse should be carefully watched for, noting both heart rate and blood pressure frequently. If signs of shock appear, intravenous fluids, plasma, blood, adrenalin-like drugs may all be used to maintain an effective peripheral circulation. It may be necessary to continue the treatment of shock for some days before the patient can be safely left without this support.

Because of these serious and too often fatal complications of poisonings which would otherwise be treated successfully, a great deal depends on the close observation of the patient and the early detection of developing complications. In this matter the nurse is of the greatest importance. A careful and readily available chart should be kept of the patient's blood pressure, heart, rhythm and respiratory rate, color and reflex activity. Often these observations may have to be noted every 15 minutes. Gradual trends may be better indicated by a graph than by any other method of charting data.

Specific Antidotes

Specific antidotes are used in cases in which the poison has been definitely identified and of course, only in the case of poisons for which there is a specific antidote. Specific antidotes are those which counteract the poison directly, or antagonize its pharmacologic action in the body. Such measures, therefore, depend on the chemical and pharmacologic nature of the poison. Unfortunately, effective specific antidotes are available for only a small proportion of poisons. In most cases, however, the eventual outcome depends more on the prompt application of the general measures than on the specific antidotes.

A few of the specific antidotes may be mentioned here. Dimercaprol (BAL) is an outstanding measure against heavy metals. It antagonizes the effects of arsenic, gold, mercury and other metals on one of the vital enzyme systems in cells. It is not useful in all types of metal poisoning, however. For barbital poisoning, picrotoxin, metrazol and amphetamine are effective physiologic antidotes. In strychnine poisoning and other types of convulsant poisons, ether, barbiturates and other depressant drugs can exert potent physiologic antagonism and patients may be saved from as much as 10 fatal doses. Physostigmine is effective in atropine poison, and vice versa. Physostigmine is also effective in curare poisoning. Atropine is an effective antagonist against mecholyl poisoning. Copper sulfate, a highly toxic material itself, is a specific chemical antidote in phosphorus poisoning. Sodium formaldehyde sulfoxalate is a specific chemical antidote for mercury poisoning but it has given way to the more effective physiologic antidote, dimercaprol (BAL). In the case of morphine poisoning, a new drug, n-allylnomorphine appears to be promising as a specific physiologic antidote. It is well to remember that most physiologic antidotes are also potent drugs in their own right, and given incorrectly, may themselves induce serious poisoning.

A very effective antidote for lead poisoning has just been introduced. The drug, commonly called EDTA but now officially named edathamil and also known as a versene, is a chelating agent, a material which literally pulls metals from its combination with the substance of the tissues and organs. It then forms a soluble compound of the metal which is less toxic and more rapidly excreted. Its usefulness in lead poisoning is already clear and it seems likely that it will also be effective in poisoning by other metals; but proof of this is not yet established.

Potassium permanganate is commonly used in alkaloidal poisoning because it destroys a great many (but not all) of them rapidly. It is important to remember that this antidote is also a toxic material and that only dilute solutions should be given orally or results may be disastrous. Precautions should be taken to insure that concentrations over 1:10,000 are not used. Dilutions should never be made haphazardly. Properly made solutions may be effective when used to wash the stomach in cases of alkaloidal poisoning.

Drugs Used in Medical Emergencies

Analeptics	Hypertensives
Anesthetics	Parenteral fluids
Autonomics	Specific antidotes
Depressants	Stimulants (heart muscle)
Electrolytes	Stimulants (vascular)
Hormones	Stimulants (respiratory)

Study Questions

1. What are considered the most urgent medical emergencies?

2. What are the nurse's responsibilities in anticipating, recognizing and meeting these emergencies?

3. To what types of secondary effects may death be due in an individual who has suffered poisoning from some drug or other substance?

4. In the treatment of poisoning, it is very important to determine the causative agent. What is the nurse's responsibility in this respect?

5. In what ways may accidental poisoning come about?

6. In the home, how may vomiting be induced most easily in the conscious patient?

7. Why would these measures be contraindicated in the unconscious patient?

8. What measures may be taken to assure adequate respiration in a patient who has taken poison?

9. What supportive measures should the nurse anticipate the need for?

10. Tabulate antidotes which may be used in various types of poisoning, such as barbiturate, heavy metals, atropine, alkaloidal, etc.

25

DIAGNOSTIC AGENTS

Drugs which are primarily used to aid in diagnosis rather than to cure or relieve symptoms constitute an important facet of pharmacology and therapeutics. Some of these are effective therapeutic agents used for what are sometimes called therapeutic tests; their therapeutic action is so specific and so dependable that a diagnosis may be made on the effect of their administration, whether they help the patient or fail. The action of ergotamine, for example, is so specific for the relief of migraine headache, that if it fails to relieve a headache, the diagnosis of migraine becomes doubtful. Such therapeutic tests are not, however, considered in this section.

The drugs that are used for diagnostic tests may be grouped into (1) dyes, (2) radio-opaque materials, (3) metabolic drugs, (4) radioactive materials, (5) sympatholytic drugs, (6) biologic and allergic materials.

Dyes

Dyes are used for three purposes: (1) to indicate and trace abnormal communications between various structures of the body; (2) to indicate areas of damage to superficial surface, such as the eye and the skin; (3) to measure blood volume.

Radio-opaque Drugs

Radio-opaque materials are used to produce shadows in the x-ray picture. X-rays penetrate the soft structures of the body, and for this reason the softer organs cannot be seen in the ordinary unaided x-ray picture. If the organ is hollow and can be filled with a material which is opaque to x-ray, the material will cast a shadow in the x-ray picture which conforms to the shape of the inside of the hollow organ. Thus, the gastro-intestinal tract is filled with

269

barium, by mouth or by rectum, and visualized in this way in the x-ray picture. Drugs may be administered by mouth which are excreted into the gall-bladder, the urinary bladder, or the pelvis of the kidney. Other radio-opaque materials may be injected into the kidney pelvis, the urinary tract, spinal canal, the uterus, the cavities of joints and the bronchial tree.

In addition, the rate with which some of these organs excrete these radio-opaque materials, may also be used as an indication of function as well as of anatomic configuration. The rate and completeness with which the gastro-intestinal tract expels the barium placed in it also indicates functional activity.

Metabolic Drugs

Metabolic materials are drugs which are normally excreted or destroyed in the body in a particular way or rate which is altered in disease. These variations from the normal may be measured and used as diagnostic tests. Thus the way a patient handles sugar may be used to test the function of his pancreas and establish the diagnosis of diabetes (sugar-tolerance test); the ability of the liver to excrete or destroy certain drugs is the basis of liver function tests; the ability of the kidney to excrete phenolsulfophlein dyes is the basis of several kidney function tests.

Radioactive Drugs

Radioactive drugs are materials which have been activated in the atomic pile so that they exhibit radioactivity. Because of this their presence can be detected with a Geiger counter and measurements can be made of rates of elimination, concentration and so forth. Radio-iodine, for example, is picked up selectively by the active thyroid gland; the rate at which it is picked up, determined with the Geiger counter, may be taken as an index of thyroid function and disease.

Sympatholytic Drugs

Sympatholytic drugs, described in detail elsewhere (page 118), antagonize or abolish the effects of epinephrine. This action may be used diagnostically to differentiate between high blood pressure of the usual variety, and that due to a tumor of the adrenal gland, called a pheochromocytoma, which causes overproduction of epinephrine. In this test the drug is given and the effects on blood pressure carefully watched.

Biologic Materials

In some infectious diseases, long after the disease has been cured, and in many allergic states, the patient's skin develops specific hypersensitivities which may be used for diagnostic purposes. Thus in the case of allergies, scratch or injection tests with allergens may be used to determine the specific offending allergen while in some infectious diseases the injection into the skin of immune substances, antitoxins, toxins and vaccines may produce specific reactions which indicate the diagnosis.

Drugs Used in Diagnosis

Allergenic Extracts   Radio-opaque materials
Adrenolytics   Serums
Antitoxins   Toxins
Dyes   Vaccines
Radioactive Drugs

Study Questions

1. Indicate examples of the various types of drugs used in diagnostic tests and specify the purpose in each case.

2. What are the nurse's responsibilities?

INTRODUCTION

The medicine prescribed is here differentiated from drugs; the medicine represents the final product of the doctor's science and the pharmacist's art. The medicine is what is given to the patient to take. The drug is the active ingredient of the medication, which also contains vehicles, flavors, emulsifying agents, diluents, solvents and coloring matter necessary to make it more palatable, more acceptable, more agreeable and perhaps, even more effective for the patient.

The nurse stands in a crucial and delicate position in the matter of the administration of the medicine. The doctor writes the order for the drug and the dose to be given, and it is the best practice to insist, wherever possible, that a written order be left. If the nurse is wise she will go over the order with the doctor before he leaves. If the doctor is wise, he will do it without being asked. In any event, at this point the doctor's responsibility in the matter of administration of the medicine ceases and that of the nurse begins.

What are the nurse's responsibilities in the giving of medication? (1) She must understand the doctor's orders. (2) She must recognize and identify the drugs prescribed. (3) She must measure the doses correctly. (4) She must give the medication on time and in the manner designated. How much this entails depends not only on what the doctor wants, but also on how the orders are left and other attending circumstances. In one case the doctor may leave an ampule representing the entire dose of the drug; the nurse needs only to open the ampule and to inject all its contents. In another case the hospital pharmacist may supply a stock bottle from which the nurse has to measure the needed amount which she must deter-

274

mine by her own calculations. In another case she may find that the drug is available under another name in her own ward medicine cabinet. In another case the drug may be prescribed in a system of measurement not used in the hospital and the nurse may have to convert the prescribed dose into the system used before she can calculate the dose to give. In still another case she may find that the written orders left by the doctor are so illegible as to leave her insecure, or that abbreviations have been used which she does not understand.

The duties of the nurse in administering medicines imply certain qualifications; namely, (1) the ability to read prescriptions and doctors' orders; (2) knowledge of synonyms of common drugs; (3) knowledge of common Latin terms and common abbreviations; (4) knowledge of the units of weights and measures used in dosage and in the translation from one system of measure to another; and (5) facility in the arithmetic of dosage calculation.

The failure of the nurse in any of these may turn out to be a serious matter for the patient; it may make the difference between a dose which is effective and one which is ineffective, or even worse, the difference between the effective dose and one which poisons him. It is for this reason that the written order is so important as a document that the proper dosage was prescribed, and it is also for this reason that it is so valuable for all concerned to have the nurse go over the written orders with the physician before he leaves the patient. Such consultation with the physician should be a routine matter, done in such a way that it neither embarrasses the physician nor leaves an impression of insecurity about the nurse; done properly it should give confidence that the nurse is taking every precaution necessary for the proper care of the patient.

26

THE PRESCRIPTION

Prescriptions are official, formal, written orders from the physician to the pharmacist directing that he take certain drugs and compound them into a medication according to certain directions. In this matter it is, in a sense a recipe, and indeed, the curious sign at the head of all prescriptions, ℞, is supposed to stand for *Recipe*, a command in Latin to the pharmacist, "Take Thou." The prescription also contains a set of orders for the nurse or whoever is handling the administration of the medication on the details of when, where, how and how much of the medicine to give. Although the nurse is rarely called on in the course of her duties to read a full and formal prescription such as the doctor writes to the pharmacist, patients often inquire about them and, in general, it is well for her and for her standing with the patient to be able to read and understand the prescription; in some situations it is essential to her duties.

There are four parts to the prescription: (1) superscription, (2) inscription, (3) subscription, (4) signature. The superscription is the symbol ℞ appearing at the top of the form. The inscription lists all the drugs, vehicles, flavors, colors, diluents, solvents, and the amounts of each. The subscription consists of the directions to the pharmacist for compounding the prescription. It tells him the kind of preparation to make and what form it should take: pills, capsules, powders, tablets, solutions, emulsions, ointments, troches, suppositories, etc. The signature consists of the specific intructions for the patient: when, where, how, how much and with what to take the medication. These instructions are to be copied by the pharmacist onto the bottle or box containing the medication. The subscription and signature are commonly written with a great many Latin abbreviations.

The prescription itself should always bear the patient's name and address. This is important for it provides a means of finding the patient, should the pharmacist discover that some error has been made in compounding the prescription. The patient's age should be indicated since it provides a check against dosage which, by error, may have been written with an adult in mind but prescribed for a child. The doctor's name, address, and phone number are always on the prescription blank so that the pharmacist may contact him should there be any question concerning the prescription. All these precautions have proved to be of practical importance for there are many instances in which a life has been saved because it was possible to contact a patient or a physician after an error had been discovered.

The modern prescription tends to be rather simple and the nurse will find fewer of the older and more complex or so-called "shot-gun" prescriptions used as time goes on. Examples of a simple prescription follows, written in English and in Latin, with the metric and the apothecary system of measure.

Dr. Joseph Smith
19 Maple Lane, Boston
Tel: BO. 1-4069

Jan. 4, 1953

John Jones   Age: 45
15 Maple Lane, Boston

℞

Chloral Hydrate	1.0 Gm.
Sodium Bromide	2.5 Gm.
Water to make	100 cc.

Mix and make solution
Label: One teaspoonful every night

Signed: Joseph Smith, M. D.

Dr. Joseph Smith
19 Maple Lane, Boston
Tel: BO 1-4069

Jan. 4, 1953

John Jones   Age: 45
15 Maple Lane

℞

Chlorali Hydrati   gr. xx
Sodii Bromidi   gr. 1
Aquae q. s. ad   ℨ iv
Misce
Sig.   One teaspoonful every night.

Signed: Joseph Smith, M. D.

27

MEDICAL ENGLISH AND LATIN

Most prescriptions are now written in English but many are still written in Latin. The nurse who does not know Latin is presented with no particular problem, for the Latin is hardly ever of such a nature that special knowledge is required. The Latin used in instructions is standardized and often written in well-known abbreviations (Table 5). The latter are so frequently used that it is essential for the nurse to know them well. The designation of drugs in Latin is no great hardship, because virtually all important drugs have identical or such closely similar names in Latin and in English that they are readily identified without any knowledge of Latin at all. It is amusing to note that the few drugs that have decidedly different names in the two languages, for the most part, are not important or potent drugs, but older drugs, flavors or oils which can be readily identified by the patient by smell or taste. For example water is *aqua*, honey is *mel*, castor oil is *oleum ricini* and whiskey is *spiritus frumenti*, while morphine, penicillin and strychnine have identical official names in Latin and English. Table 6 lists some of the drugs which have different names in the two languages. A quick glance will indicate how few of these represent important drugs. Virtually all new drugs are now given identical names in Latin and English.

Names of Drugs

A source of some confusion lies in the variety of names one drug may have. One of these is the chemical name which may be a long and complex one, usually used only with new drugs. There is also the official name which may be the chemical name if it is

Table 5—Common Latin Words and Abbreviations

Abbreviation	Latin	English Meaning
āā.	Ana	Of each
a.c.	ante cibus	Before meals
Ad	Ad	To, up to
Add	Adde	Add
Ad lib.	Ad libitum	At pleasure
Agit.	Agita	Shake or stir
Alb.	Albus	White
Alt. hor.	Alternis horis	Every other hour
Ante	Ante	Before
Aq.	Aqua	Water
Aq. bull.	Aqua bulliens	Boiling water
Aq. dest.	Aqua destillata	Distilled water
Aq. ferv.	Aqua fervens	Warm water
Aq. frig.	Aqua frigida	Cold water
Bis	Bis	Twice
B.i.d. or b.d.	Bis in die	Twice daily
c̄	Cum	With
Cap.	Capiat	Let the patient
Caps.	Capsule	Capsule
Cleriter	Celeriter	Quickly
Chart.	Chartula	A medicated paper or powder
Coch. mag. or amp.	Cochleare magnum or amplum	A tablespoonful
Coch. med.	Cochleare medium	A dessertspoonful
Coch. parv.	Cochleare parvum	A teaspoonful
Col.	Cola	Strain
Comp. or co.	Compositus	Compound
D.t.d. no.	Dentur tales doses no.	Give—such doses
D., det.	Da, detur	Give, let be given
Dil.	Dilutus	Dilute
Disp.	Dispensa	Dispense
Divid	Divide	Divide
El.	Elixir	Elixir
Ex	Ex	From
Ext.	Extractum	Extract
Et	Et	And
E.m.p.	Ex modo praescripto	After the manner prescribed
ft. or F.	Fac, fit, fiat, fiant	Make, let be made
Filt.	Filtra	Filter
Fl.	Fluidus	Fluid
Flext.	Fluidextractum	Fluidextract
Gm.	Gramma	Gram
gr.	Granum	Grain
Gt. or gtt.	Gutta	A drop
Hor. som or h.s	Hora somni	At bedtime
In	In	In, into
Inj.	Injectio	An injection

Table 5—continued

Abbreviation	Latin	English Meaning
Liq.	Liquor	A liquor
M.	Misce	Mix
Mag.	Magnus	Large
Mass.	Massa	A mass
M. dict.	Modo dictu	As directed or prescribed
Non rep.	Non repetatur	Do not repeat
No.	Numerus	Number
O.	Octarius	A pint
O.D.	Ocular dexter	Right eye
Omn. hor.	Omni hora	Every hour
Omn. man or o.m.	Omni mane	Every morning
o.n.	Omni nocte	Every night
Opt.	Optimus	Best
os	os	Mouth
O.S. or O.l.	oculus sinister or laevus	Left eye
O.U.	Oculus uterque	Each eye
P.e.	Partes aequales	Equal parts
Per	Per	Through
Pil.	Pilula	Pills
Post cib. or p.c.	Post cibo	After eating
P.r.n.	Pro re nata	According to circumstances
Pulv.	Pulvis	A powder
q.d.	quaque die	Every day
q.i.d.	quarter in die	Four times a day
q. 1 (2,3) h.	Quaque una (dua, tres) hora	Every 1 (2,3) hours
q.s.	Quantum sufficat or satis	A sufficient quantity
℞	Recipe	Take
Rept.	Repetatur	Let it be repeated
s̄	Sine	Without
s.o.s. or si. op. sit.	Si opus sit	If it is needed
S.A.	Secundum artem	According to art
ss.	Semiss	A half
Sig. or S.	Signa	Label or let it be imprinted
Sol.	Solutio	Solution
Solv.	Solve	Dissolve
Spir, or Sp.	Spiritus	Spirit
Stat.	Statim	At once
t.i.d.	Ter in die	Three times a day
Tab.	Tabella	Tablet
Tal.	Talis	Of such, like this
Tr., Tinct.	Tincture	Tincture
Trit.	Tritura	Triturate
ung.	Unguentum	Ointment
Ut. Dict.	Ut dictum	As directed
Vin.	Vinum	Wine

Table 6—Names of Some Common Drugs in Which English and
Latin Names Are Not Similar

English	Latin
Alcohol	Spiritus Vini Rectifactus
Almond Oil	Oleum Amygdalus
Beef	Caro
Castor Oil	Oleum Ricini
Chalk	Creta
Coal Tar	Pix Carbonis
Cod Liver Oil	Oleum Morrhuae
Corn Oil	Oleum Maydis
Cottonseed Oil	Oleum Gossypii Seminis
Ginger	Zinziber
Iron	Ferrum
Lard	Adeps
Larkspur	Delphinium
Lead	Plumbum
Lime	Calyx
Linseed	Linum
Liver	Hepar
Mercury	Hydrargyrum
Mustard	Sinapis
Orange Oil	Oleum Aurantii
Ox Bile	Fel Bovis
Peanut Oil	Oleum Arachidis
Peppermint	Mentha Piperita
Pine Tar	Pix Pini
Raspberry	Rubus
Rhubarb	Rheum
Silver	Argentum
Smallpox Vaccine	Vaccinum Variolae
Soda Lime	Calx Sodica
Spearmint	Mentha Viridis
Starch	Amylum
Water	Aqua
Wax	Cera
Whiskey	Spiritus Frumenti
Wool Fat	Adeps Lanae
Yeast	Saccharomyces

short, or an acceptable abbreviation, if it is long and cumbersome.
Official names are usually followed by some designation such as
U.S.P., N.F. or N.N.R. These are the names doctors and nurses
should use. The next category is that of trade names, to which there
is no limit. Those may be designated with the sign, ®. Finally, there
are sometimes many synonyms without any particular standing.

For example, desoxephedrine and *d*-N, alpha-dimethyl-phenthyl-
amine hydrochloride are chemical names for metamphetamine hydrochloride, U.S.P. The latter is the official name which is the one
that should be used by doctors and nurses. Amphedroxyn hydrochloride, desoxyn hydrochloride, dexoval, efroxine, norodin and
syndrox are some of the trade names for the same material. Since
this is a Pharmacopoeial drug, it is under government control and
there is no reason why any one particular product has any superiority over another. Thus the six trade-named drugs all indicate
the same material. As a matter of fact, they may even be produced
by the same manufacturer and sold by him to the various drugs
houses which in turn give the drugs their own name before distribution to the confused medical public.

It may be noted that in this text, although the official names of
drugs are usually given, in the interest of ready understanding a
much better known proprietary name may sometimes be used
instead.

28

WEIGHTS AND MEASURES

Matters have not been made simpler for either the doctor or nurse by the fact that two systems of measure are currently used in dosage. The older system, the apothecary system, is used only in this country and Great Britain. It is the system of grains and minims, of drams and ounces. Its only virtue is that it is well known in these parts. It is cumbersome and difficult to handle when precise measurmeent of dosage is required. It remains with us only because it is well known and because it is so difficult to change habits, either personal or national, once they are well established. The older physicians, especially, who were taught only the apothecary system in medical school, resist all attempts to change over into a better system. Nurses who were trained years ago also have great difficulty in making the shift. The nurse, however, is in an entirely different position from the doctor, for he can choose what he wants to use, while the nurse must operate in the system of measurement the doctor decides to use. Although the apothecary system is slowly being discarded, she must learn all about it and know how to handle it with facility. The British imperial measure involves only minor differences in the larger quantities.

The alternate and preferred system of measurement is the metric system. It is used in all fields of science because it makes calculations simpler and lends itself to accuracy. It is used exclusively in all modern practice outside the United States and Great Britain. Its use in medicine simplifies matters for everyone, the doctor, the pharmacist and the nurse. All that is needed to establish it is a determination on the part of physicians to discard the old for the far better metric system. There is the possibility that the U.S.P. will use the metric system exclusively in future editions. This will be a powerful stimulus to the general use of that system of measurement of drugs.

Apothecary System

The apothecary system can be compared with the English system of money (pennies, shillings, pounds and guineas), which confuses Americans when they go to England because nothing seems to go evenly into anything else. The system of money in this country, which is really a decimal system, is much easier to work with. This is so because it is comparable to the metric or decimal system, in which each unit is a tenth of the next larger unit; thus we have cents (hundredths), dimes (tenths) and dollars (units). It is in fact a decimal system of money and was chosen because we are practical about money matters. The apothecary system of weights and measures is just as illogical and just as cumbersome as the English monetary system.

In the apothecary system, Roman numerology is used except for fractions smaller than one-half. Fractions are written in Arabic (common) numerals. The Roman numerals are written in small letters rather than in capitals as usually taught in school:

½ = ss	8 = viii
1 = i	9 = ix
2 = ii	10 = x
3 = iii	20 = xx
4 = iv	30 = xxx
5 = v	40 = xl
6 = vi	50 = l
7 = vii	

Numerals larger than 50 (1) are rarely used. Some physicians may use a "j" instead of a final "i," e.g., they will write 3 as iij, rather than iii. In writing in the apothecary system the numbers always follow the abbreviations of the units of measure, instead of preceding them as in the metric system, thus 10 grains is written gr. x.

The smallest unit of weight is the grain. It is to be distinguished from the similarly sounding gram, a unit of the metric system which is 15 times as large. It is important that every precaution be taken to prevent confusion between the two, since such an error might result (and has resulted) in giving a patient 15 times as large a dose as intended. For this reason the abbreviations are made distinctly different, thus gr. for grain and Gm. for gram. The capitalization of the "G" in gram brings it into sharp contrast with the small "g" in grain.

The dram, occasionally spelled drachm, and abbreviated ʒ (or dr.) is the next unit in size. It is equal to 60 grains. The largest practical unit of weight in dosage prescription is the ounce, abbreviated ℥ (or oz.). It is equal to 8 drams and 480 grains. The pound of the apothecary system is equal to 12 ounces and is rarely used in prescriptions.

Table 7—Apothecary System Equivalents

1 pound (lb.)	=	12 ounces
1 ounce (℥)	=	8 drams
1 dram (ʒ)	=	60 grains (gr.)
1 pint (O)	=	16 fl. ounces
1 fl. ounce (℥)	=	8 fl. drams
1 fl. dram (ʒ)	=	60 minims (♏)

There is no connection between the units of weight and of liquid measure. Liquids are measured according to their volume in prescriptions made up in this country and Great Britain. This is to be distinguished from the practice on the European continent where both solids and liquids are weighed and, therefore, liquid or volume measure is not used at all.

The smallest unit of liquid measure is the minim, abbreviated m or ♏. The next unit is the fluid dram, abbreviated fl.ʒ, or now commonly designated in exactly the same way as the dram of weights, ʒ. The fluid dram is equal to 60 minims. The largest common unit in prescription writing is the fluid ounce, abbreviated fl.℥ or ℥. It is equal to 8 drams and 480 minims. The pint, abbreviated O, is equal to 16 ounces.

As far as possible when amounts are expressed in the apothecary system it is done in the largest permissible single unit, thus an amount equal to one dram and 30 grains is usually expressed as a dram and a half (ʒiss) rather than ʒi gr. xxx.

Metric or Decimal System

The metric or decimal system is the system of science and by far the easier of the two to manipulate. Most of the difficulty with it comes from the fact that this system is taught as a deviation from an established system. It may make the approach to the metric system more acceptable if it is pointed out that in this system, common or Arabic numerals are always used, fractions are never used and the arithmetic is far simpler. As a matter of fact, this is such a universal practice that it can be assumed that the metric system is used when abbreviations for units of measure are not indicated, and the quantities are written in Arabic numerals.

The meter is the fundamental unit of the metric system and gives it its name. In the measurement of drugs, however, the meter is never used, and the basic units of measure are grams for solids and cubic centimeters for liquids. It may be pointed out again that in Europe, though the metric system of dosage is used, liquid measure is never applied and that all drugs, both liquid and solid are weighed. In this country, when the metric system is used, solids are always weighed and liquids are always expressed in terms of volume. There is no deviation from this rule. Arabic numerals are used in the metric system. Thus when writing in the metric system it is not essential to indicate the unit of measure; if a solid drug is referred to, grams will be used; if it is a liquid, cubic centimeters will be assumed.

Table 8—Metric System Equivalents

1.0 kilogram (Kg.)	= 1000 grams
1.0 gram (Gm.)	= 1000 milligrams (mg. or mgm.)
1.0 liter (L.)	= 1000 cubic centimeters (cc. or ml.)

In the measurement of solids, doses are expressed as grams, abbreviated Gm., or milligrams. Doses may be expressed entirely in terms of grams and its decimal portion. Thus a 5 grain aspirin tablet which is approximately equal to 300 mg. is usually designated as 0.3 Gm. On the other hand, small doses, 0.1 Gm. or less, are often expressed in terms of milligrams. Thus a dose of demerol may be expressed as 100 mg. instead of 0.1 Gm; the dose of morphine as 10 mg. rather than 0.01 Gm.; the dose of nitroglycerin as 0.4 mg. instead of 0.0004 Gm. Note that the decimal point is preceded by a cipher (0) in all cases in which there is no whole numeral. Some physicians find that it leads to better and more accurate practice to use a long vertical line instead of a period (.) to represent the decimal point. Thus they write 0/3 rather than 0.3 Gm. It may be pointed out for the sake of completeness, and also to understand the writing of foreigners, that in many European countries a comma is used instead of a point. Thus a dose may be written 0,3 instead of 0.3 Gm.

There is a definite relationship between the liquid and solid measure in the metric system; the gram is the weight of a cubic centimeter of water. The smallest unit of liquid measure is the cubic centimeter, abbreviated cc. Doses smaller than one cubic centimeter are expressed as decimal fractions of the cc. In some texts the abbreviation, ml. (milliliter or one-thousandth of a liter), may be seen, but as far as the nurse is concerned there is no difference between the ml. and the cc.

In the metric system the only units larger than the gram and the cubic centimeter which are usually encountered are the liter which is equal to 1000 cc. and approximately 1 quart, and the kilogram, equal to 1000 Gm. and approximately 2.2 pounds.

Conversion

It is often necessary for the nurse to translate from one system to the other. Facility in such translation can come only with practice. A few equivalents are listed in table 9.

A list of approximate and rounded equivalents of doses which are commonly used may be found in table 10; those not used in dosage forms are not included. The values given in the table are sufficiently accurate and easy to handle; it would be well to memorize these equivalents since calculation can then be done with ease, chances for error will be decreased and the final dosage will be accurate. The slight margin of error introduced by the rounding of the numbers has already been considered by the Pharmacopeial Com-

Table 9—Metric and Apothecary System Equivalents

Metric	Apothecary Equivalent
1 mg.	$^1/_{64}$ grain
1 Gm.	15½ grains
1 Kg.	2.2 lbs.
1 cc.	16¼ minims
1 Liter	1 quart
Apothecary	Metric Equivalent
1 grain	0.065 (65 mg.)
1 dram	3.9 Gm.
1 ounce	31 Gm.
1 minim	0.064 cc.
1 fluid dram	3.7 cc.
1 fluid ounce	29.6 cc.

Table 10—Rounded Dosage Equivalents for Metric and Apothecary Systems

Weights				Liquid		
Apothecary	Metric			Apothecary	Metric	
gr. $^1/_{200}$	0.0003	Gm. or	0.3 mg.	ℳ i	0.06	cc.
gr. $^1/_{100}$	0.0006	Gm. or	0.6 mg.	ℳ ii	0.12	cc.
gr. $^1/_{60}$	0.0001	Gm. or	1.0 mg.	ℳ iii	0.2	cc.
gr. $^1/_{50}$	0.0012	Gm. or	1.2 mg.	ℳ v	0.3	cc.
gr. $^1/_{30}$	0.002	Gm. or	2.0 mg.	ℳ viiss	0.5	cc.
gr. $^1/_{12}$	0.005	Gm. or	5.0 mg.	ℳ x	0.6	cc.
gr. $^1/_8$	0.008	Gm. or	8.0 mg.	ℳ xv	1.0	cc.
gr. $^1/_4$	0.015	Gm. or	15.0 mg.	ℳ xxx	2.0	cc.
gr. $^1/_2$	0.03	Gm. or	30.0 mg.	℥ i	4.0	cc.
gr. i	0.06	Gm. or	60.0 mg.	℥ ii	8.0	cc.
gr. iss	0.1	Gm. or	100.0 mg.	℥ ss	15.0	cc.
gr. ii	0.12	Gm.		℥ i	30.0	cc.
gr. iii	0.2	Gm.		℥ ii	60.0	cc.
gr. v	0.3	Gm.		℥ iv	120.0	cc.
gr. viiss	0.5	Gm.		℥ vii	180.0	cc.
gr. x	0.6	Gm.		℥ viii	250.0	cc.
gr. xv	1.0	Gm.		quart	1000.0	cc.
gr. xxx	2.0	Gm.				

mittee. It is permissible and the problem may, therefore, be dismissed without further discussion.

Conversion from one system to another is often necessary and is, unfortunately, conducive to errors. The best way to avoid errors is to memorize the equivalents so well that calculation is rarely required. There are some rules which one should also learn to enable conversion from the metric to the apothecary system and vice versa:

Rule: To convert milligrams to grains divide by 60.
Example: Convert 15 mg. to grains
(1) 15÷60=¼ grain

Rule: To convert grains or minims to grams or cubic centimeters divide by 15.
Example: Convert 30 grains to grams
(1) 30÷15=2 Gm.

Rule: To convert drams to grams or cubic centimeters multiply by 4.
Example: Convert 4 drams to cubic centimeters
(1) 4×4=16 cc.

Rule: To convert ounces to grams or cubic centimeters multiply by 30.
Example: Convert 2 ounces to cubic centimeters
(1) 2×30=60 cc.

Rule: To convert grains to milligrams multiply by 60.
Example: Convert ¼ grain to milligrams
(1) ¼×60=15 mg.

Rule: To convert grams or cubic centimeters to grains or minims multiply by 15.
Example: Convert 2 Gm. to grains
(1) 2×15=30 grains

Rule: To convert grams or cubic centimeters to drams divide by 4.
Example: Convert 16 cc. to drams
(1) 16÷4=4 drams

Rule: To convert grams or cubic centimeters to ounces, divide by 30.

Example: Convert 60 cc. to ounces

(1) 60÷30=2 ounces

It should be noted that the approximate values are used here; these are quite satisfactory for all purposes to which a nurse may be required to apply such calculations.

If an answer comes out in a decimal or fraction, such as 24.72 cc., it is permissible to round out the number to the nearest whole number, 25 cc. if the error introduced by such a procedure does not exceed 10 per cent of the total dose. Thus it would not be permissible to round off 22.43 to 25 because the error introduced would be too large.

Study Questions

1. Express the following as grams: (a) 0.2 mg., (b) 50 mg., (c) 0.1 Kg., (d) 6 mg., (e) 15 mg., (f) 0.1 mg., (g) 300 mg., (h) 2 Kg.

2. Using numbers and symbols, convert the following to their approximate equivalents: (a) gr. ½, (b) ℥iii, (c) 300 mg., (d) 0.015 Gm., (e) 120 cc., (f) 0.6 Gm., (g) 20 mg., (h) ℥viii, (i) gr. ⅙, (j) 45 cc., (k) 0.0002 Gm., (l) gr. ¹/₁₅₀, (m) 8 mg., (n) ℳ xlv, (o) ℥ss, (p) ℨxv, (q) 32 mg., (r) 0.06 Gm.

29

MEDICAL ARITHMETIC

Some facts of simple arithmetic may well be reviewed, for facility and accuracy in arithmetic are essential to the nurse. Without this skill she is insecure about one of her critical functions, the calculation of the dose she gives her patient. Much has been made of the intricacies of the processes of dosage calculation but this is entirely unwarranted. The relative simplicity of dosage calculation arises from the uniformity of size of doses of drugs prescribed. Doses tend to fall into three ranges: (1) from 5 to 15 grains, (2) from ⅛ to 1 grain and (3) from $^1/_{50}$ to $^1/_{200}$ grain, and their metric equivalents. There is the added simplifying feature that doses are usually given in rounded numbers, such as 5 or 10 grain, ½ or ¼ grain, $^1/_{100}$ or $^1/_{200}$ grain; these are simple figures which are easy to deal with.

In the metric system doses tend to group themselves as follows: (1) from 0.25 mg. to 5 mg., (2) from 10 mg. to 100 mg. and (3) from 250 mg. to 1 Gm.

The processes in calculation are of the same order as everyday household calculations; nothing more than simple addition, subtraction, multiplication and division. The aspects of arithmetic which are reviewed will be just as simple as the problems in dosage calculation which occur in actual practice.

Fractions

It is our experience that fractions give more trouble, and hence require more review than any other aspect of arithmetic. Dangerous mistakes have been made by people who do not have a clear understanding of fractions; this is an especially critical area because drugs which are prescribed in fractions of grains are, as a rule, the more potent and toxic drugs. There have been instances in which a patient was given a dose of $^1/_{50}$ of a grain of nitroglycerin under the impression that it was half, rather than twice as large as gr. $^1/_{100}$. There are also cases in which a gr. $^1/_{100}$ tablet was broken in half under the impression that it provided gr. $^1/_{50}$. Of course, it actually provided only a dose of gr. $^1/_{200}$.

For a better understanding of fractions it might be helpful if the meaning of the word were better understood. If you "fracture" or "fraction" something you break it into parts. "Fractions" are merely numbers which represent the grouping of such parts of the whole number. The fraction, as it is represented numerically gives two pieces of information: (1) It denotes the number of equal parts into which the whole has been broken. In the common fraction this information is provided by the bottom figure, the denominator. (2) It counts (enumerates) the number of equal parts which have been combined to make up the particular fraction. In the common fraction this is indicated by the upper figure, the numerator.

Common Fractions

Thus, in the common fraction, $\frac{3}{4}$, the denominator (4) denotes that the whole has been broken into 4 equal parts, and the numerator (3) enumerates the 3 parts which have been combined to make up the fraction. For example, when we speak of a period of time as three-quarters of an hour, we are really indicating that we have broken a whole hour into 4 equal parts (or quarters) and that we are considering the portion of the hour comprised of 3 of these quarters.

Decimal Fractions

The decimal fraction gives the same kind of information as the common fraction. In the decimal fraction the denominator is always 10 or a multiple of 10. For example, in our monetary system which uses decimals, $0.75 is identical with 75/100 of a dollar. The numerator is 75 and the denominator is 100.

Fractions as Ratios

Fractions are also a means of expressing ratios. When we say that three-fourths of the beds in a hospital are occupied we compare one quantity with another: occupied beds with all the beds in the hospital. The ratio is 3:4. The ratio of 3:4 can, of course, apply to a larger hospital as well as a smaller one; 15:20 or 45:60 or 75:100 all boil down to the same ratio of 3:4 or ¾ when written as a fraction.

The significance of a 100 bed hospital in our example is that it automatically shows its occupancy in per cent (per hundred). The expression 75% has no other meaning than 75:100 or 75/100 or 0.75. Naturally, all the other hospitals (the 20 bed, 60 bed, 100 bed hospitals of our example) also have a 75 per cent occupancy. The ratio concept is used to *compare* quantities, not to give information about sizes or magnitudes.

Reduction of Fractions

As already indicated the same value for a ratio may be expressed in an unlimited variety of equal numerical forms; i.e., 1:2, 2:4, 3:6, 4:8, 5:10, etc. When these are expressed as common fractions it is self-evident that $\frac{1}{2} = \frac{2}{4} = \frac{3}{6} = \frac{4}{8} = \frac{5}{10}$. This is because the ratio or relationship between the numerator and the denominator is the same in each case, one-half. The simplest expression in the series is ½ but it does not differ in the slightest from the largest, $\frac{5}{10}$, or any other fraction in which the numerator is half of the denominator, for example $\frac{5000}{10,000}$.

Rule: The value of a fraction is determined by the ratio of the numerator to the denominator. As long as this ratio is not disturbed, the value of the fraction remains the same regardless of how the magnitude of the numerator and denominator is altered.

The expression of a particular fraction in another numerical form is known as reduction. Reduction may be required for simpler expression or for easier calculation. It never alters the actual value of the fraction, it merely expresses it in another form. The two types of reduction are descending or simplification and ascending or expansion.

Descending Reduction

This form of reduction is usually called simplification. In the process, fractions are reduced to the point of simplest expression in which the numbers in numerator and denominator are as small as possible. The ratio, however, remains unchanged.

Rule: For descending reduction: (1) Divide the numerator and the denominator by the largest number which will go evenly into both. (2) The quotient of the division in each case provides the numerator and denominator of the reduced fraction.

An alternate method is as follows: (1a) Divide the numerator by a small number which will go evenly into each. (2a) Continue this with the quotient in each case until it is no longer possible to divide both by the same number no matter how small. (3a) The remaining quotients provide the numerator and denominator of the reduced fraction.

Example: Simplify $^{12}/_{24}$.

Calculation:

(1) $$\frac{12 \div 12}{24 \div 12} = \frac{1}{2}$$

(1a) $$\frac{12 \div 2}{24 \div 2} = \frac{6}{12} \quad \frac{6 \div 3}{12 \div 3} = \frac{2}{4} \quad \frac{2 \div 2}{4 \div 2} = \frac{1}{2}$$

Ascending Reduction

For addition and subtraction it may be necessary to expand fractions so that all the denominators are the same. A common example of such expansion is the expression of $\frac{1}{2}$ as $^{5}/_{10}$.

Rule: For ascending reduction: (1) Multiply the numerator and the denominator by the same number. (2) The products provide the numerator and denominator of the expanded fraction.

This process may be continued endlessly as long as the precaution is taken to multiply both numerator and denominator by the same number.

Common Denominator

The ascending reduction of fractions is used mainly in addition and subtraction of fractions. The process involves the reduction of all fractions in a series with different denominators to fractions

with the same denominators. In most instances of dosage calculation the fraction with the largest denominator provides the common
denominator.

The qualification for a common denominator is that it must be
evenly divisible by the denominators of all the other fractions. The
rule given below is adequate for cases of dosage calculation in
which it is necessary to determine a common denominator.

Rule: To determine a common denominator: Multiply the incompatible denominators (those that are not evenly divisible, one
into the other).

Example: Determine the common denominator of ⅓ and ⅛.
Calculation:

(1) 3×8=24, the common denominator.

When the common denominator is determined all fractions in
the series must be reduced to the common denominator.

Rule: For ascending reduction of fractions to a common denominator: (1) Divide the denominator of the fraction into the common
denominator. (2) Multiply the numerator of the fraction by the
quotient of the division. (3) The product is the numerator of the
fraction over the common denominator.

Example: Reduce ¾ to the common denominator 8.
Calculation:

(1) 8÷4=2
(2) 2×3=6
(3) The reduced fraction with common denominator=⁶/₈.

Mixed Numbers

Mixed numbers are fractions which are larger than 1, usually
expressed in the form of a whole number plus a fraction. An hour
and a half, written 1½ hours, is an example of a mixed number.
When a fraction is larger than 1 it may be preferable to reduce it to
a mixed number, especially for the expression of the answer in a
dosage calculation. It is far better form, for example, to speak of
the total dose of a drug as 7½ grains than ¹⁵/₂ grains.

Rule: To reduce a fraction larger than 1 to a mixed number: (1) Divide the numerator by the denominator. (2)* The whole number in the quotient is the whole number of the mixed number. (3) The remainder in the quotient is the numerator of the fraction of the mixed number. (4) The denominator of the fraction remains the same.

Example: Express $^{18}/_4$ as a mixed number.

Calculation:

(1) $18 \div 4 = 4$ plus a remainder of 2
(2) the whole number is 4
(3) the numerator of the fraction is 2
(4) the denominator of the fraction is 4
(5) the answer is $4\frac{2}{4}$ or $4\frac{1}{2}$

Arithmetic Operations with Fractions

Up to this point we have covered the basic concepts necessary to deal with fractions in the same way as whole numbers. In order to continue the demonstration that operations with fractions are simple procedures which we handle in our daily life we shall continually refer to the face of the clock and fractions of the hour.

Looking at the face of the clock we see that its circumference is divided. In some cases there are 12 large numerals which divide the face into 12 equal divisions or hours. Some clock faces also have 60 equal divisions, each representing $^1/_{60}$ of the hour or a minute. Clock faces with modern design may have only 4 numerals which break the circumference into 4 equal parts or quarters representing 3 hour intervals when the hour hand points to them and 15 minute or quarter hour intervals when the minute hand points to them.

Consider how easily you handle these fractions of the clock face, how you add the quarters and halves, subtract them, multiply and divide them. Bear in mind that the fractions used in dosage calculation are of the same order as the fractions of the hour you handle

---

*The easiest way to understand why step 2 is carried out is to examine the example. Since 4 quarters are equal to 1, the number of times 4 may be divided into 18 is equal to the number of whole units in $^{18}/_4$. The remainder represents the number of quarters in excess of these whole numbers.

so well. Most fractional doses are halves, quarters and eighth grain doses.

Addition

Addition with fractions is essentially the same as with whole numbers. One may find, for example, that it takes one-quarter of an hour to bathe and one-quarter of an hour to dress. At once we know that the sum of the times is two-quarters of an hour (or one-half hour). The process of addition in this case involved the addition of the numerator while the denominator remained unchanged.

This process cannot, however, be carried out in exactly this way in the case of the addition of fractions with different denominators. When the denominators are not the same, a common denominator must be determined and the fractions reduced before the addition of fractions can be completed as in the case just given. If in going somewhere, the ride in the train takes one-half hour and the ride in the bus takes one-quarter of an hour, the total time spent in travel equals three-quarters of an hour. Note that the denominator of the fraction, one-half, has disappeared in the process. What was unconsciously done in this operation was first to convert the one-half hour to 2 quarters, and then to add the 2 (quarters) to the 1 (quarter) to total 3 (quarters).

Rule: To add fractions: (1) If there are no common denominators convert all fractions to a common denominator. (2) Add the numerators. (3) The sum is the numerator of the sum of the fractions. (4) The denominator of the sum is the common denominator. (5) When possible the resulting fraction may be reduced.

Example: Add ½ grain and ⅛ grain.
Calculation:

(1) the common denominator is 8; $\frac{1}{2} = \frac{4}{8}$
(2) $4+1=5$
(3) the numerator of the sum is 5
(4) the denominator remains 8
(5) the sum of the fractions is ⅝ (which cannot be reduced)

Rule: To add mixed numbers the whole numbers and fractions are totaled separately.

Example: Add 12½ grains and 7½ grains.

Calculation:

$$(1) \quad \begin{array}{r} 12 \; \frac{1}{2} \\ + 7 \; \frac{1}{2} \\ \hline 19 \; ^2/_2 \end{array}$$

(2) By reduction $^2/_2 = 1$, and the total of the mixed numbers, therefore, equals 20.

Subtraction.

Subtraction of fractions is also essentially the same as with whole numbers. If one person can do a job in a quarter of an hour while another takes one-half hour for the same job, it is clear that the first person takes one-quarter of an hour less than the second. The mental operations involved in obtaining this result were as follows: ½ was converted to $^2/_4$ and ¼ was subtracted from it, leaving the remainder of ¼. The fractions were converted to a common denominator and the numerators were subtracted while the denominator remained unaltered.

Rule: To subtract fractions: (1) Convert the fractions to a common denominator. (2) Subtract the numerator of the subtrahend from the numerator of the minuend. (3) The remainder is the numerator of the new fraction. (4) The denominator remains the common denominator. (5) If it is possible the remainder should be reduced.

Example: Subtract ⅛ grain from ½ grain.

Calculation:

(1) ½ is reduced to the common denominator, $^4/_8$
(2) 4—1=3
(3) the numerator of the remainder is 3
(4) the denominator of the remainder is 8
(5) the answer is ⅜ which cannot be further reduced

Check: To check, add the remainder and the subtrahend; if the total equals the minuend the check is satisfactory.

Example: Check the preceding example.

Calculation:

(1) ⅜ (remainder) +⅛ (subtrahend)=⁴/₈=½ (minuend)

In subtraction with mixed numbers, as in the case of addition, the whole numbers and fractions are treated separately. If, however, the fraction in the minuend is smaller than the fraction in the subtrahend, it may be necessary to borrow a unit from the whole number, reducing it by 1, and increasing the value of the fraction correspondingly. This is, of course, the same process which is carried out in the subtraction of whole numbers when one of the figures of the minuend is smaller than that of the subtrahend in the same column.

Example: Subtract 2⅞ from 9⅜.

Calculation:

(1) clearly ⅞ cannot be subtracted from ⅜
(2) convert 9⅜, therefore, to $8+^8/_8+^3/_8=8^{11}/_8$
(3) proceed as in subtraction

$$8 \ ^{11}/_8$$
$$-2 \ ^7/_8$$
$$\overline{6 \ ^4/_8} \quad \text{by reduction}=6½}$$

Multiplication

Multiplication with fractions is much more of an everyday experience than most of us realize. If it takes you half an hour to drive somewhere, you know that you can get half way there in one-quarter of an hour. In this mental calculation you have actually multiplied ½ (of the hour) with ½ (of the way there). In this process the numerators were multiplied and the denominators were multiplied, and the answer was the fraction made up of the products. Note that in this process the value of the fraction tends to become small, usually smaller than either the multiplier or the multiplicand. This is so because multiplication with fractions means fractionation, that is, making things smaller.

Rule: To multiply fractions: (1) Multiply the numerators. (2) Multiply the denominators. (3) The product of the numerators over that of the denominators is the product of the multiplication of the fractions. (4) If possible, the product may be reduced.

Example: Multiply ¾ grain by ½.

Calculation:

(1) $3\times1=3$, numerator of the answer

(2) $4\times2=8$, denominator of the answer

(3) $\frac{3}{8}$, the answer, cannot be further reduced

Check: Divide the answer by the multiplier; if the quotient is equal to the multiplicand, the check is satisfactory.

Example: Check the preceding example.

(1) $\frac{3}{8}\div\frac{1}{2}=\frac{3}{4}$

Note: In the case of multiplication between a whole number and a fraction the whole number is changed to a fraction by setting it over the denominator, 1. For example to multiply $5\times\frac{1}{2}$, change the 5 to $\frac{5}{1}$ and proceed as above.

Division

In one of the examples given above, a girl took half an hour to do a job which another girl did in a quarter of an hour; one knows at once that the slower girl took twice as long as the quicker girl to do the job. This conclusion comes as the result of the mental division of $\frac{1}{4}$ (of an hour) into $\frac{1}{2}$ (of an hour). The result of this division is 2. Note that exactly the opposite kind of result is obtained as in the case of multiplication, namely that the answer is larger than the original figures. An analysis of what was done in this case reveals that a smaller fraction was fitted into a larger fraction, hence the result will be larger than the dividend.

In our above example the division of $\frac{1}{4}$ into $\frac{1}{2}$ results in the answer 2 because there are $\frac{2}{4}$ in $\frac{1}{2}$. That is to say, in the division of fractions two processes are required: (1) the conversion of the fractions to a common denominator and (2) the division of the numerators. In the rule given below, by a trick (step 1), the common denominators are determined and cancelled out in one operation. These steps will, therefore, for the purposes of simplicity, be eliminated and the common denominator will not be mentioned in the rules which follow.

Rule: To divide with fractions: (1) Invert the divisor and proceed as in multiplication. (2) Multiply the numerators. (3) Multiply the denominators. (4) The product of one over the other is the answer. (5) If possible, the answer may be reduced.

Example: Divide ¾ grain by ½.

Calculation:

(1) invert ½=²/₁
(2) 3×2=6
(3) 4×1=4
(4) ⁶/₄, the answer, =1½

Check: To check a division multiply the quotient by the divisor; if the product equals the dividend the check is satisfactory.

Example: Check the preceeding example.
(1) ⁶/₄×½=⁶/₈=¾

Decimals

The decimal is nothing more nor less than a fraction written in a special system of notation in which the fraction and the whole number are separated by a decimal point. It is the normal and proper system of notation and as a consequence the system lends itself to simple and accurate calculation.

The basis of the decimal system lies in our system of numbers. These run in groups of 10, from 0 to 9, which are arranged in vertical columns to make these groups, 0 to 9, 10 to 99, 100 to 999 and so forth. The numbers in each succeeding column of figures have 10 times the magnitude of the numbers with a smaller number of figures, for example, 1, 10, 100, 1000. Conversely, reduction of the number of figures reduces the magnitude of numbers by one-tenth, for example, 8000, 800, 80 and 8. Thus the addition of a cipher results in multiplication by 10 and the removal of a cipher is the same as division by 10.

The decimal is a continuation of this phenomenon into fractions. In this system all fractions are reduced to tenths or its multiples, one-hundredths, one-thousandths and so forth. The decimal fraction starts at the right of the decimal point; the first figure is tenths (0.5 is five-tenths), the second is hundredths (0.05 is five-hundredths), the third is thousandths (0.005 is five-thousandths). Thus each move to the right of the decimal point represents a division by 10 and each move to the left, multiplication by 10, exactly as we have seen with whole numbers.

It is to be noted that any number of ciphers may be added to the right of the last figure after the decimal point without altering the value of the number in the slightest. Thus 1 and 1.0000000 and 1.56 and 1.560000 are equal. On the other hand it must be emphasized that the position of the decimal point represents a critical area for mistakes. By the nature of things in the decimal system an error in one decimal place represents a error ten-fold in magnitude, and error in two decimal places represents a hundredfold error. The magnitude of the error which may result from the incorrect placing of the decimal point is usually far greater than any which may develop as the result of an error in arithmetic processes. The rules for the placement of the decimal point in calculations must, therefore, be carefully observed.

Arithmetic Operations with Decimals

Decimal fractions, whether larger or smaller than one, are dealt with exactly the same way as whole numbers. The only feature requiring special attention is the position of the decimal point; the rules for this are somewhat different in the case of each operation. The basic arithmetic processes, as they apply to decimals will be briefly considered.

Addition

The only precaution is to align the decimal points vertically. Add the columns from right to left in the usual way, making no special change at the decimal point except to indicate it. Matters may be made simpler for some by filling in the spaces to the right of the decimal point so that all numbers are of the same length:

$$
\begin{array}{lll}
12.5 & & 12.500 \\
.05 & \text{or} & .050 \\
.006 & & .006 \\
\hline
12.556 & & 12.\,556
\end{array}
$$

Subtraction

The same precautions apply as in addition, namely the correct alignment of the decimal points before starting the subtraction, and the indication of its position in the remainder, directly under the points in the column. Empty spaces may be filled with ciphers if desired:

12.5		12.50
− 1.05	or	− 1.05
11.45		11.45

Multiplication

The process is exactly the same as with whole numbers and the only issue concerns the placement of the decimal point. Multiplication proceeds as usual without regard to decimal places. After the product is obtained the position of the decimal point must be determined.

Rule: To determine the position of the decimal point in a product of multiplication: (1) Add the number of decimal places in the multiplier and multiplicand. (2) Count off an equal number of figures from the right of the product and place the decimal point between this figure and the next one on its left.

Example: Multiply 1.25 and 1.5.

Calculation:

(1) $125 \times 15 = 1875$
(2) the sum of the decimal places is 3
(3) the decimal point must, therefore, lie between the third and fourth figures from the right, namely, 1.875

Division

Here too the arithmetic is the same as with whole numbers. The position of the decimal point may be determined on its completion.

Rule: To determine the position of the decimal point in a quotient: (1) Count the number of figures to the right of the decimal point in the divisor and remove. (2) Move the decimal point in the dividend an equal number of places to the right. (3) Place the decimal point in the quotient directly under the decimal point in the dividend.

Example: Divide 15.555 by 0.5

Calculation:

(1) $15555 \div 5 = 3111$

(2) there is 1 decimal point in the divisor

(3) move the decimal point in the dividend from 15.555 to 155.55

(4) the decimal point in the quotient will fall below it=31.11

Common Fractions Expresed as Decimal Fractions

It is often a practical matter in calculations to convert a common fraction to a decimal fraction. In many examples this conversion is done automatically:

$$^2/_5 = {}^4/_{10} = 0.4 \qquad \text{or} \qquad ^3/_4 = {}^{75}/_{100} = 0.75$$

Rule: To express a common fraction as a decimal fraction divide the denominator of the fraction into its numerator. This procedure is actually a short cut for dividing the denominator into the "decimal denominator" (10,000 or 1000 and so on) and then multiplying the numerator with the quotient obtained.

Example: Express ¼ as a decimal fraction.

Calculation:

(1) $1 \div 4 = 0.25$

Percentage

To determine any percentage problem it is necessary to know only two of the following three items: (1) the percentage, (2) the total amount, (3) the amount making the percentage.

Examples of this type of problem will be given in the section on solutions which constitute the major problems of percentage in dosage calculation.

Common Fractions Expressed as Percentage

We have already seen how common fractions may be expressed as decimal fractions. As the nurse may be called upon to make this calculation she may also have to convert common fractions into percentage.

Rule: To express a common fraction as a percentage: (1) Divide the denominator of the fraction into its numerator. (2) If the quotient has more than two figures to the right of the decimal point(more than hundredths), place the decimal point between the hundredth and the thousandth.

Example: Express ⅝ as a percentage.

Calculation:

(1) 5.000÷8=.625
(2) .625=62.5%

PROCEDURES IN DOSAGE CALCULATION

Medicine is available in (1) fixed forms, (2) prescription bottles and (3) stock bottles. Each presents different problems in the measurement of the proper dose.

Fixed Forms

Fixed forms of medicine are forms in which the amount for each separate dose has been measured by the pharmacist or manufacturer and made into a unit which can be kept and taken individually. These include such pharmaceutic preparations as ampules, perles, capsules, pills, tablets, papers, troches, suppositories, lozenges. When a fixed form has been prescribed all one needs to do in those cases in which the dose is *larger* than the amount in each form is to determine the amount in each fixed form, and to give the proper number of them. Thus if the dose of a sulfonamide drug prescribed is 1.5 Gm. and the tablets contain 0.5 Gm. each, the patient should be given 3 such tablets. On the other hand, the dose prescribed may be *smaller* than the amount in the fixed form. There are some tablets which are grooved or scored in halves or in quarters for precisely such circumstances. In such a case, the tablet properly broken along the groove provides an accurate fraction on the tablet and supplies the dose prescribed. When no such provision for fractioning a fixed form is made, it is bad practice to attempt it.

Dosage Problem: The number of fixed forms in a dose.

Explanation: The number will be equal to the number of times the amount in the total dose exceeds the amount of drug in the fixed form.

Rule: To determine the number of fixed forms in a dose: (1) Divide the amount of drug in the fixed form into the dose prescribed. (2) The quotient is the number of fixed forms which will supply the dose.

Example: Administer 2.0 Gm. sulfadiazine to a patient, 0.5 Gm. tablets being provided.

Calculation:

(1) $2.0 \div 0.5 = 4$

(2) 4 tablets are required

Hypodermic injections may have to be made from tablets which do not correspond to the dose prescribed. For example, an injection of gr. ⅛ morphine sulfate may be ordered but the tablet provided may contain gr. ¼. It is at once clear that one-half of the tablet is needed, since gr. ¼ is twice as large as gr. ⅛, but the problem is how to divide the tablet in half accurately. The simplest solution to this problem is to dissolve the tablet in a small amount of water or saline, to draw it up into a hypodermic syringe and to expell half of the solution. The remaining solution will contain gr. ⅛ morphine sulfate. Precautions to maintain sterility must, of course, be taken in all steps of the procedure.

Dosage Problem: To obtain a dose from a hypodermic tablet which exceeds the dose prescribed.

Explanation: Make a solution from the tablet and take a portion which contains the dose.

Rule: To obtain a dose from a tablet which exceeds the dose: (1) Divide the dose ordered into the dose provided. The quotient represents the number of times the tablet exceeds the dose needed. (2) Dissolve the tablet in a small amount of water or saline and bring this up to a convenient amount by further dilution in the syringe, usually between 0.25 and 0.5 cc. or 15 to 30 minims. Select a value which is easily divisible by the quotient in step 1.* (3) Divide the quotient of step 1 into the amount of fluid in the syringe. (4) Keep the amount of this value and expell the remainder. (5)

---

* It will often simplify calculation by choosing a value for dilution in step 2 which is evenly divisible by the quotient of the calculation in step 1. In the example, 15 minims is chosen for the volume because it is evenly divided by 1½.

Bring up to a satisfactory volume for injection with proper dilutent.

Example (apothecary system): Administer a hypodermic injection of gr. ⅛ morphine sulfate being provided with a gr. ¼ tablet.

Calculation:

(1) ¼÷⅛=1½

(2) dissolve tablet and bring up to 15 minims in syringe; mix

(3) 15÷1½=10

(4) retain 10 and expel 5 minims from the syringe; this contains gr. ⅛

(5) dilute with water or saline to 15 minims

Example (metric system): Administer a hypodermic injection of 10 mg. being provided with a 25 mg. tablet of morphine sulfate.*

Calculation:

(1) 25÷10=2.5

(2) dissolve tablet and bring up to 0.25 cc. in syringe; mix

(3) 0.25÷2.5=0.10

(4) retain 0.10 cc. and expel 0.15 cc.; this contains 10 mg. morphine sulfate

(5) dilute with water or saline to 0.25 cc.

Prescription Bottles

The prescription bottle contains a liquid medication which is usually prescribed in doses measured in household utensils. In any case in which the dose is prescribed in terms of a household utensil, the drugs involved must be of such a nature that the widest latitude in dosage is permissible. Such measurement may never be used in cases in which accurate dosage is essential, for it is impossible to achieve accuracy with any ordinary household measuring device. It is well to bear in mind that the teaspoon, which is the commonest

---

* Such problems occur infrequently in institutions in which the metric system is used because most of the hypodermic tablets now manufactured in this country are put up in apothecary dosage. In addition, hospitals using the metric systems frequently supply such drugs in stock solutions.

household article used for measuring liquid medications, varies widely in its capacity. This depends, on the one hand, on how the spoon is filled, for someone with a steady and cautious hand may fill a teaspoon so that it contains twice as much as one filled by someone with a tremor. A second factor is the design of the spoon; some teaspoons hold as much as 7 cc., others only about 4 cc. Such variation in content applies equally to other household measuring devices. The physician is, of course, aware of this when he prescribes his medicine. When he thinks that accuracy is a matter of importance, he either uses a fixed form or he orders the use of an accurate measuring device such as a special dropper or a graduate.

Household articles frequently used for measuring liquid medications are listed below with their approximate capacities:

1 teaspoonful	=	4 to 6 cc.	or ℨ i
1 dessertspoonful	=	8 cc.	or ℨ ii
1 tablespoonful	=	15 cc.	or ℥ ss
1 wineglassful	=	50 to 60 cc.	or ℥ ii
1 tumblerful	=	250 cc.	or ℥ viii

The common medicine dropper provides a drop of variable size depending on the opening at the bottom and the viscosity of the medication. In situations in which accuracy is not important the drop is taken as being equal to 1 minim or 0.05 cc. A calibrated dropper, really a kind of pipet, is used when accuracy is essential; here fluid is measured in actual amount and not drops. The calibrated dropper which looks like an ordinary dropper merely delivers the medication in drops, but it measures it in actual amount and is useful and convenient for measuring small amounts of fluid. In all cases in which drops are used as the unit of measure the attempt should be made to use the same dropper at all times.

Stock Bottles

Stock bottles contain solutions or suspensions of drugs, frequently parenteral preparations, in quantities larger than the single dose. Stock bottles are used because they reduce the cost of drug preparation. The content of the stock bottle may be sterile and the bottle of the multiple-dose type with a special rubber stopper so that the drug can be removed without opening the bottle and exposing its contents to contamination. A common example is the insulin bottle.

The labeling of the stock bottle may indicate its content in either of two ways: (1) the amount of drug per cubic centimeter or minim of solution, or (2) the concentration of the solution, i.e. a percentile or ratio solution.

Drug per Fluid Unit

Labels which indicate the amount of drug present in each fluid unit make calculations relatively simple.

Dosage Problem: The number of fluid units in a dose taken from a stock bottle labeled in terms of drug per fluid unit.

Explanation: The number will be equal to the number of times the dosage exceeds the amount of drug in each fluid unit.

Rule: To obtain a dose from a stock bottle labeled in drug per fluid unit: (1) Divide the amount of drug in each unit into the total dose. (2) The quotient is the number of fluid units which will provide the dose.

Example (metric system): Administer a dose of 100,000 units of penicillin from a bottle labeled 500,000 units per cc.

Calculation:

(1) $100,000 \div 500,000 = 0.2$

(2) 0.2 cc. provides the dose

Example (apothecary system): Administer a dose of gr. ¼ morphine sulfate from a bottle containing Magendie's solution which contains gr. xvi in each fluid ounce.

Calculation:

(1) $\frac{1}{4} \div 16 = \frac{1}{64}$

(2) $\frac{1}{64}$ ounce provides the dose; this is equal to minims viii

Solutions Expressed as Ratios

Such solutions are virtually always used for washes, irrigations and the like, never for providing individual doses for injection. They do not, therefore, present a problem in dosage calculation.

Percentile Solutions—Metric System

In instances in which the drug in a stock bottle is expressed in percentage concentration of the drug the nurse is given more work in dosage calculation. Fortunately, however, this is rarely done. The problem is considerably simpler in the metric than the apothecary system.

Dosage Problem: The amount of solution, expressed as a percentage, which contains a dose.

Explanation: Translate the percentage into content per fluid unit and proceed as above for the stock solution.

To determine the amount of drug per cubic centimeter proceed on the basis that each cubic centimeter weighs 1 Gm. or 1000 mg. Since a 1 per cent solution contains 1 part of drug per 100 parts of solvent, each 100 mg. of solution will contain 1 mg. of drug, and 1 cc. (1000 mg., i.e., 10 times the weight) will contain 10 mg. More dilute and more concentrated solutions will contain correspondingly more or less drug per cubic centimeter. On this basis table 11 was constructed; it is well to memorize it.

Table 11—Percentage Equivalents of Milligrams of Drug per Cubic Centimeter

Per cent	mg. drug per cc.
0.1	1
1.0	10
2.0	20
3.0	30
4.0	40
5.0	50
10.0	100

Rule: To obtain a metric dose from a percentile solution: (1) Determine the amount of drug per cubic centimeter. (2) Divide this into the dose of drug. (3) The quotient is the number of cubic centimeters which contains the dose.

Example: Administer a 100 mg. dose of demerol from a 2 per cent stock solution.

Calculation:

(1) a 2 per cent solution contains 20 mg. per cc.
(2) 100÷20=5
(3) the dose is contained in 5 cc. stock solution

Percentile Solutions—Apothecary System

Since the metric system is a decimal system it is closely allied to percentage, a fact which makes calculation easy. In the apothecary system, however, decimal relationships do not exist as part of the system and calculations are, therefore, relatively more difficult. To simplify matters, it is assumed that there are 500 (actually there are 480) minims or grains to the ounce. On this basis 5 grains will make 1 ounce of a 1 per cent mixture. For each per cent in the apothecary system there are 5 grains or minims to the ounce. Table 12 is based on this premise.

Table 12—Percentage Equivalents of Grains or Minims per Ounce

Per cent	grains or minims per ounce
1	5
2	10
3	15
4	20
5	25
6	℥ ss per ounce
10	50 grains or minims per ounce
12	℥ i per ounce

Percentile stock solutions are rarely used for individual doses in the apothecary system, but occasionally an apothecary dose must be obtained from a percentile solution. The basis of calculation is essentially the same as in the metric system, and one method of solution is to translate the dose into the metric system and to proceed as already shown. The second method is to translate the concentration of the solution into terms of apothecary doses per apothecary fluid unit and then to follow a procedure essentially the same as for metric dosage.

Rule: To obtain an apothecary dose from a percentile solution:

(1) Determine the amount of drug per ounce. (2) Divide the amount per ounce by 500; this is the amount per minim. (3) Divide the dose by amount per minim. (4) The quotient is the total dose in minims; convert to a convenient unit.

Example: Administer gr. viiss of caffeine sodium benzoate from a stock bottle containing a 10 per cent solution.

Calculation (first method):

(1) gr. viiss=0.5 Gm. or 500 mg.

(2) 10 per cent solution contains 100 mg. per cc.

(3) 500÷100=5

(4) 5 cc. or ℥ 1¼ provides the dose

Calculation (second method):

(1) 10 per cent solution contains 50 grains per ounce

(2) 50÷500=¹/₁₀

(3) 7½÷¹/₁₀=75

(4) 75 minims or ℥ 1¼ provides the dose

Study Questions

1. You. as a nurse, have the orders for medication shown in Column I. You find that the labels on the various bottles read as indicated in Column II. Indicate in Column III how much you would give in the form supplied.

Column I	Column II
Cediland 0.0006 Gm., I. V.	0.4 mg./cc.
Aqueus penicillin 250,000 U., I. M.	500,000 U./cc.
Heparin 0.05 Gm., I.V.	10 mg./cc.
Thiomerin 210 mg., s.c.	0.14 Gm./cc.
Aminophyllin 200 mg., I. V.	0.25 Gm./10 cc.
Morphine sulfate 0.015 Gm.	15 mg./0.5 cc.
Dicumarol 0.25 Gm., p. o.	100 mg./capsule

2. You have an order for codeine phosphate 0.06 Gm., p.o. The bottle of tablets provided is labeled gr. ss. How would you prepare the medication?

3. Prepare a subcutaneous medication, morphine sulfate gr. ⅛ from hypo tablets labeled gr. ⅙.

31

PROCEDURES IN THE PREPARATION
OF SOLUTIONS

Drugs which are available in solutions may be injected, diluted, applied to the skin and mucus surfaces, and easily varied in dos: These are the advantages of having a drug in solution. The disadvantages are that solutions have a taste, they tend to deteriorate more rapidly than solid preparations and they are relatively bulky.

The physical nature of solutions is that they represent the perfect mixture of drug and diluent; every portion of the solution has exactly the same proportion of drug and vehicle. The solutions which are made up for use in medicine are available in percentile, ratio and unit volume forms. This is the order in which they will be discussed in this chapter.

Percentile Solutions

Solutions are often made in terms of percentage concentration. As already explained, the percentage is the ratio of the number, expressed as the percentage, and 100. In the case of the percentile solution, the percentage represents the number of parts of drug in each 100 parts of solution. The following three elements enter all percentile problems: (1) the percentage, (2) the amount of drug and (3) the total amount of solution. Any problem in dosage calculation can be solved with two of these three items. The following types of problems may arise: (1) to determine the amount of drug needed to make a stated amount of a particular concentration, (2) to determine the volume necessary to make a stated percentage solution of a given amount of drug and (3) to determine the percentage concentration of a solution with a stated volume and drug content.

315

Metric System

Percentile solutions should, wherever possible, be calculated in the metric system because it provides a solution that is easy to calculate and make up, and less liable to error. These advantages are not to be found when using the apothecary system.

Problem: To make a percentile solution.

Explanation: Dissolve 1 Gm. of drug in 100 cc. or Gm. diluent for each per cent.

Rule: To make a percentile solution: (1) Divide the total volume ordered by 100. This gives the amount of drug necessary to make a 1% solution. (2) Multiply the percentage ordered by the amount of drug necessary for a 1% solution. (3) The product is the number of grams or cubic centimeters for the required volume.

Example: Make 600 cc. of a 5 per cent dextrose solution.

Calculation:

(1) 600÷100=6

(2) 5×6=30

(3) dissolve 30 Gm. of dextrose in 600 cc. solution

The problem is solved in exactly the same when less than 100 units are ordered.

Example: Make 25 Gm. of a 2 per cent salicylic acid ointment in petrolatum.

Calculation:

(1) 25÷100=0.25

(2) 2×0.25=0.5

(3) 0.5 Gm. salicylic acid mixed with 25 Gm. petrolatum

Another problem in percentage calculation is how much of a particular percentage can be made with a given amount of drug.

Rule: To determine the amount of solution: (1) Divide the percentage into the amount of the drug. This gives the number of hundreds of cc. of solution which can be made up. (2) Multiply the quotient by 100. (3) The product is the total volume.

Example: How much 5 per cent solution can be made with 10 Gm. salt?

Calculation:

(1) 10÷5=2

(2) 100×2=200

(3) 200 cc.

The remaining problem in percentile calculation is the determination of the percentage of a solution when the amount of drug and the volume are known.

Rule: To determine the percentage of a solution: (1) Divide the total volume into the amount of drug. This gives the fraction of 100% concentration. (2) Multiply the quotient of step 1 by 100. (3) The product is the percentage.

Example: What is the percentage concentration of a dextrose solution in which 10 Gm. dextrose is dissolved in 50 cc. water?

Calculation:

(1) 10÷50=0.2

(2) 0.2×100=20

(3) 20 per cent solution

Apothecary System

The basis of percentile calculation in the apothecary system is the fact that there are approximately 500 grains (or minims) to the ounce. It follows, therefore, that a 1 per cent solution contains 5 grains (or minims) to the ounce (i.e., 1 grain for each 100 grains) and that a percentage can be made up by dissolving 5 grains (or minims) for each per cent per ounce.

Rule: To make a percentile solution: (1) Multiply the number of per cent by 5. (2) Multiply the product of step 1 by the number of ounces. (3) The product is the number of grains or minims to be dissolved in the total volume.

Example: Make up 8 ounces of a 5 per cent sugar solution.

Calculation:

(1) 5×5=25

(2) 25×8=200

(3) dissolve 200 grains of sugar in 8 ounces water

Ratio Solution

As already explained, a ratio is a comparison of magnitudes. In certain forms of medication, especially dilute solutions, the concentration of the drug may be expressed as a ratio. It is common, for example, to speak of a solution of acriflavine used for the irrigation of the bladder as a 1:10,000 solution. This tends to emphasize the extent of the dilution of the solution, and from that point of view it represents a safety factor. The expression means, in terms of its dilution, that 1 part of the drug was dissolved in 10,000 equally sized parts of the diluent, in this case, water. For purposes of making a solution designated in this way, it is usually simpler to convert the ratio into a percentile expression and then to proceed as is the case of the percentile solutions. Table 13 shows the percentage equivalents of common ratios.

Table 13—Ratios and Percentage Equivalents

Ratio	Percentage
1:25	4
1:50	2
1:100	1
1:1000	0.1
1:2000	0.05
1:5000	0.02
1:10,000	0.01

Problem: To convert a ratio to percentage.

Explanation: Since percentage is merely the expression of a ratio in which one of the magnitudes is 100, it is necessary only to convert the parts of diluent to hundreds.

Rule: To convert a ratio to percentage: (1) Divide the second quantity in the ratio into 100. (2) Divide the first quantity in the ratio into the quotient of step 1. (3) The result is the percentage represented by the ratio.

Example: Convert the ratio solution 1:2000 to a percentile form of expression.

Calculation:

(1) $100 \div 2000 = .05$
(2) $.05 \div 1 = .05$
(3) $.05\% = 1:2000$

Unit Volume Solutions

Solutions may also be prepared to indicate the dosage per unit volume. In preparing the type which is labeled according to the amount in each cubic centimeter, or in each minim, dram or ounce, the calculations are relatively simple.

Problem: To prepare a solution containing a stated amount per fluid unit.

Explanation: The total amount of drug needed is determined by the amount of drug in each fluid unit and the total number of fluid units.

Metric System

Rule: To prepare a solution containing a stated amount of drug per cubic centimeter: (1) Multiply the total number of cubic centimeters by the dose in each cubic centimeter. (2) The product is the total amount of drug to be dissolved in the total volume.

Example: Make up 100 cc. of a salt solution containing 100 mg. per cc.

Calculation:

(1) $100 \times 100 = 1000$

(2) dissolve 1000 mg. (1.0 Gm.) in 100 cc. water

Apothecary System

Rule: To prepare a solution containing a stated amount of drug per fluid dram: (1) Multiply the total number of drams by the dose in each dram. (2) The product is the total amount of drug to be dissolved in the total volume.

Example: Make up 4 ounces of a sugar solution containing gr. v per dram.

Calculation:

(1) 4 ounces = 32 drams, hence $32 \times 5 = 160$

(2) dissolve 160 grains (approximately ℥ iiss) in ℥iv solution

Dilution of Solutions

Sometimes a more dilute solution has to be made from a concentrated stock solution. It may be pointed out that while it is possible to do the reverse, namely to make more concentrated solutions out of weaker ones by either boiling off water or adding more drug, neither of these procedures is permissible.

Problem: To dilute a solution.

Explanation: The amount of dilution necessary will correspond to the number of times the original solution exceeds the desired solution in strength. The following must be known: (1) nature of diluent, (2) concentration of the stock solution, (3) concentration desired, (4) amount of diluted solution needed.

Rule: To dilute a solution: (1) Divide the concentration of the desired solution into that of the stronger solution. (2) Divide the quotient of step 1 into the amount of diluted solution needed. (3) The quotient is the amount of stock solution to be used. (4) The difference between the quotient and the total volume needed is the amount of diluent needed.

Calculations are the same in both apothecary and metric systems, but far more simple in the metric system·

Example: Make up 500 cc. of a 2.5 per cent solution from a 10 per cent stock solution of sucrose.

Calculation:

(1) $10 \div 2.5 = 4$

(2) $500 \div 4 = 125$

(3) 125 cc. stock solution required

(4) $500 - 125 = 375$ cc. of diluent necessary

Solutions from Tablets

Sometimes the nurse is called upon to make a solution from a tablet which contains more drug than is necessary for the needed amount of solution. The problem and the solution, in many ways, resembles that of giving a hypodermic dose when the tablet provided exceeds the dose prescribed.

Problem: To make a solution from a tablet which contains more than the necessary amount of drug.

Explanation: Make a stronger solution than called for and dilute a portion or make a larger amount of desired solution than is necessary.

Rule: To make a solution from a tablet containing more drug than necessary: (1) Follow the rule for dilution of concentrated solutions, or (2) follow the rule for percentile solutions.

Example: Make up 10 cc. of a 1 per cent saline solution from a 0.3 Gm. tablet.

Calculation (method 1):

(1) dissolve the 0.3 Gm. tablet in 10 cc.

(2) by calculation this turns out to be a 3 per cent solution

(3) by calculation this requires 3 to 1 dilution to make 1 per cent

(4) dilute 3⅓ cc. of concentrated solution to 10 cc. of water

Calculation (method 2):

(1) by calculation 0.3 Gm. makes 30 cc. of 1 per cent solution

(2) hence, dissolve the tablet in 30 cc. water

(3) retain 10 cc. and discard or save the remaining 20 cc. solution

Saturated Solutions

Making a saturated solution is properly the duty of the pharmacist; it is rarely that of the nurse. A saturated solution is one which has reached the highest point of concentration possible with the drug in question, the solvent not being able to dissolve any more of the drug. The exact amount necessary to make a saturated solution varies with each drug and depends not only on how soluble it is but also on the temperature of the diluent. This information may be found in a chemical or pharmaceutic handbook. If this data is not available proceed along these lines: add a large amount of drug to the total amount of solvent, mix and allow to stand at room temperature for from several hours to a day. The solution should be agitated from time to time and, if the drug tolerates it without deterioration, it may be gently warmed. If all the drug dissolves, more should be added, for it may be that still more drug will be dissolved into the solution; hence it is not certain that a saturated solution has been made until it has been determined that the solvent will not dissolve any more drug. The process must, therefore, be repeated until added drug no longer dissolves but remains at the bottom of the solution. The clear solution is then poured or filtered off.

This is a most unsatisfactory way of proceeding and it is far better and less time consuming, to determine from a table just how much drug is required to make up a given amount of saturated solution and to proceed with that information.

Study Questions

1. Prepare ℨvi of 2 per cent sodium perborate for a mouth wash.

2. Prepare 1 liter of a 0.025 per cent solution of benzalkonium chloride.

3. How much ½ per cent solution can be made from ℨiv of cresol?

4. Prepare 250 cc. of a 5 per cent cresol solution from a 10 per cent solution.

5. Prepare 6000 cc. of a 1:3000 solution of potassium permanganate using tablets labeled 0.2 Gm.

6. Change the following to percentages: (a) 1:2000, (b) 1:50, (c) 1:40.

7. Change the following to ratios: (a) 10 per cent, (b) 0.25 per cent, (c) 0.02 per cent, (d) 0.1 per cent.

32

ADDENDUM: THE USE OF TRANQUILIZERS

The "tranquilizer" is a relatively recent addition to therapeutics. Though its meaning is by no means clear, there is already a long list of drugs to which the name is applied, and their use has spread like wildfire. While there are reports of death and disaster resulting from tranquilizers, there are also newspaper accounts of their sale on the black market and their illegal use for "kicks." The medical and social problem created by these drugs is a serious one and is growing.

Definition

Although the term, "tranquilizer," is unsatisfactory from the scientific and the therapeutic points of view, substitute designations, such as ataractic and calmative, are equally unsatisfactory. There is no uniformity in usage of the terms in the literature. Since "tranquilizer" is the most common term now, it will be used here.

A tranquilizer is meant to describe a drug that, by whatever pharmacologic action, relieves anxiety without perceptible depression of mental acuity, reaction time, or physical skill. It is a drug to relieve nervous tension, yet safe for the patient who continues to pursue a dangerous occupation, who drives a car or crosses the street in traffic, who is involved in skilled or intellectual work.

This highly particularized action of tranquilizers is in contrast to the sedative action of barbiturates, which act as general depressants and are likely to be associated with a degree of drowsiness, depression of mental acuity, and interference with intricate physical activity.

It remains to be proven that any drug can provide what the tranquilizer is said to accomplish. Given in larger than usual doses, the tranquilizers depress all the expressions of mental and physical

323

activity, despite the implication in their definition that they do not do this. There are some who question whether there is any such pharmacologic action as tranquilization and whether the results attributed to tranquilizers cannot also be achieved with the older sedative drugs in well-regulated dosages.

Meanwhile, new tranquilizers appear at a rapid rate, making the problem of final evaluation more difficult. Until actions, uses, and dangers are thoroughly explored, it would be realistic to consider tranquilizers as drugs being used for a particularized therapeutic aim that have a high potential for trouble and should not be used without trained medical supervision and clear medical indication.

Types of Tranquilizers

Almost all of the drugs that are presently being sold as tranquilizers were originally used or examined because of other pharmacologic properties. As a result, the total action of tranquilizers in the patient tends to be complex, their evaluation difficult, and their dangers varied. The drugs now available may be divided into the following categories:

(1) Rauwolfia derivatives   (3) Mephenesin-like drugs
(2) Phenothiazine derivatives   (4) Benzhydrol derivatives
                        (5) Miscellaneous

Rauwolfia Derivatives

Rauwolfia was introduced into American therapeutics for the treatment of hypertension. The crude material contains a mixture of principles, most of which appear to have similar if not identical pharmacologic actions. The best known of these principles is reserpine, well known also under a host of proprietary synonyms. More recently, another principle, rescinnamine (Moderil®), has been receiving attention.

Experience with the crude material and the purified extracts has indicated that the predominant action in hypertension is probably that of central depression. Patients with hypertension who benefited from the use of a rauwolfia material not only had a lowering of blood pressure but also appeared calmer; there were some patients in whom the blood pressure was unaffected but who, nevertheless, had their anxieties allayed. It seems probable, therefore, that the major if not the only action of the drug in hypertension is on the anxiety state. While an action on blood vessels can be demonstrated in the laboratory, this action is relatively feeble and seems to be of small clinical importance. As a result of the observations in hypertension, rauwolfia was used for its effect on anxiety as such. Its use for psychologic effects in patients without hypertension now exceeds that in hypertension.

Phenothiazine Derivatives

The first in this group of tranquilizers was chlorpromazine (Thorazine®) which belongs to the antihistaminic drugs. Investigators found it to be an exceedingly weak antihistamine but, when they looked for another use, chlorpromazine proved to be the most potent anti-emetic agent available. It was introduced into medicine thereafter until the introduction of muscle relaxants and antihistamines. The toxicity of phenothiazine, however, is to the investigation of the drug as a tranquilizer; this is now the outstanding use of chlorpromazine.

Chlorpromazine is a phenothiazine derivative. Phenothiazine itself is not new to medicine; about 25 years ago it was introduced as a urinary tract antiseptic and quickly withdrawn because of serious toxic effects. No phenothiazine derivative was used in medicine thereafter until the introduction of muscle relaxants and antihistamines. The toxicity of phenothiazine, however, is inherent in the structure of all its derivatives now used as tranquilizers and antihistamines; in spite of small chemical alterations they retain a relatively high toxic potential. It is not surprising that untoward effects, some of them serious, have been reported, especially after chlorpromazine—probably because it is longest in use. Although recently there has been a downward trend in the use of chlorpromazine this has more than been made up by the introduction of new tranquilizers, chemically closely related to chlorpromazine and, presumedly, having the same potential for harm, among them prochlorpromazine (Compazine®); pecazine (mepazine, Pacatal®); promazine (Sparine®); promethazine (Phenergan®).

Mephenesin-like Compounds

Some years ago, mephenesin (Tolserol®), available also under many other proprietary names, was introduced as a relaxant to be used in conditions in which, as in Parkinson's disease, there is excessive skeletal muscle spasm. Only large doses of mephenesin produced such relaxation, sometimes only when it was given intra-venously. Together with the muscle relaxation, there often was sedation, even somnolence, and relief from anxiety. There were many disadvantages to mephenesin, and its use is diminishing.

More recently, a mephenesin-like drug, meprobamate, was introduced. Known under the trade names of Miltown® and Equanil®, this tranquilizer is perhaps the one most widely used, certainly by the lay public without medical supervision. The indications are that meprobamate differs little from mephenesin in action. At the time of this writing, still another drug of this group, phenaglycodyl (Ultran®), was introduced.

Benzhydrol Derivatives

These drugs with sedative or tranquilizing actions that are less clearly defined than the actions in the preceding groups include hydroxyzine (Atarax®), azacyclonal (Frenquel®), meclizine (Bonamine®), chlorcyclizine (Perazil®).

Miscellaneous

Other drugs, whose actions as tranquilizers are not yet clearly defined and which are not related to the drugs above or to each other, include glutethimide (Doriden®), ectylurea (Nostyn®), methyprylon (Noludar®), ethychlorovynol (Placidyl®).

Actions and Uses

When tranquilizers are used for their tranquilizing action only, they may still be a source of trouble because of their other actions. Furthermore, in larger doses, all tranquilizers will induce somnolence. At best, tranquilization is a matter of relative dosage and, as already stated, it may be that this is the only difference between tranquilization, sedation, and hypnosis.

Psychiatric Uses

The tranquilizers have provided a means for examination of patients with severe neuroses and psychoses and have thereby stimulated psychiatric research. Tranquilizers have simplified the care of psychiatric patients, especially the more disturbed ones, so that problems of custodial care have been reduced, and the use of force and restraints has become rare. The drugs, finally, have benefited many seriously psychotic patients to such an extent that the need for institutionalization has been reduced. Many such patients can now be treated while living at home, while others are restored to their homes sooner—able to take care of themselves and to bear normal social and communal responsibilities.

These drugs *do not cure* psychiatric disorders. The patients although still ill or even disturbed, through the depressant action of the drugs, become better able to cope with the ordinary problems of everyday life. How well they will, as a group, cope with extraordinary problems of life remains to be determined.

It is clear that the drugs exert a diffuse depressant action; patients become less agitated and less anxious, slower to respond to normal stimuli, and slower to react abnormally. Considerable study is now under way to determine how it is that these drugs accomplish effects that seem to be superior to the depressant action of barbiturates.

Doses used for psychiatric patients tend to be large and often are associated with somnolence or sluggishness. Since the patients are under trained supervision, the potential for danger, however, is very small.

Medical Uses

Tranquilizers are used in general medicine to allay a wide variety of common anxiety expressions and even psychosomatic symptoms, from "nervousness," insomnia, and skin rashes to hypertension. Compared with the use of the drugs in psychiatry, the difference is not in quality as much as in quantity. In general medical care the attempt is made to alleviate anxiety of patients without producing physical or mental sluggishness; because of this use the drugs acquired the designation of tranquilizers. This pharmacologic effect is more a matter of dosage than of choice of drugs. It is interesting that one drug in this group was originally advertised as a non-barbiturate *sedative* and later as a *tranquilizer*, the only difference being in the size of the tablet, which was smaller for tranquilizing than for sedation. This constitutes recognition, by a drug manufacturer at least, that the significant difference between tranquilizers and sedatives is that of dosage.

Toxic and Dangerous Effects

When tranquilizers are used in psychiatric cases, observation by the physician is usually close and large doses are used with relative safety. In the medical case, however, the physician's supervision tends to be cursory, and the possibility of dangerous and uncontrolled drug reaction is greater. The dosage must be carefully graded to produce only the effect desired; since there is a wide range of individual sensitivity to these drugs, each patient should be carefully watched.

The tranquilizers are all relatively new; as a result, we know even less about their toxic actions than about their therapeutic potential. Even so, there is already a long list of serious difficulties that have developed through the use of these drugs. Without stating which of the tranquilizers has been implicated in each case, there have been deaths due to accidental overdosage as well as deaths from depression of bone marrow and from perforated ulcers. Serious skin rashes, convulsions, liver disorders, gastrointestinal disturbances, and allergic reactions have followed the use of these drugs. Strangely enough, there have also been severe psychologic disturbances. Persons who had been mentally normal have become manic or seriously depressed. Some have attempted suicide; occasionally with success. For some mental patients the drugs have made matters worse. One study of case records of 8200 patients reports that every other patient suffered a toxic reaction while taking a tranquilizer—an extremely high incidence.

Addiction

The matter of addiction to the tranquilizers has not yet been settled. Any drug that provides an escape from the difficulties of life presents a hazard of psychologic addiction or habituation. Since tranquilizers seem to provide such an escape for some people, the drugs should be considered and handled as potentially addictive until the question is settled.

INDEX

For detailed information about individual drugs consult the latest edition of DRUGS IN CURRENT USE, published in January of each year. DRUGS IN CURRENT USE is a comprensive alphabetical listing of drugs under their official and proprietary names as well as of pharmacologic and therapeutic groups of drugs.